LAHLEKILE
A Twentieth Century Chronicle of Nursing in South Africa

I0130423

Doreen Merle Foster

"One million people commit suicide every year"
World Health Organisation

LAHLEKILE

Published by:
Chipmukapublishing
PO Box 6872
Brentwood
Essex
CM13 1ZT
United Kingdom

www.chipmunkapublishing.com

ISBN 1-904697-52-6

DEDICATION

LAHLEKILE is dedicated to the memory of Quintin Foster who was completely and utterly proud of anything I did.

LAHLEKILE

Doreen Merle Foster

PREFACE

The South African nursing experience over 90 years has been adequately documented and may be found on the shelves of public libraries; university libraries and hospital libraries as well as between the pages of "struggle literature" such as CRITICAL HEALTH.

This book does not attempt academic analysis per se, rather is it an authentic oral and written account of the experiences, which shaped the careers of black* nurses. The sample of respondents was picked at random across the country, as time and private purse allowed. They were assured anonymity in that only first or nicknames would be used as a rule, except where a surname carries historical significance.

In 1994, when the winds of change blew democracy across the political landscape, the South African nursing profession too was gusted along the road of revolution. It was no longer a question of whether change would come, but when. Nonceba Lubanga in her chapter "NURSING IN SOUTH AFRICA" has given a detailed account of the struggle of black nurses, referring to them as "the unsung heroes of the African Struggle in South Africa." [1:51]

This book will put a human face to that titanic struggle. It is written plainly so that people outside of the academic and medical world can appreciate the violation of human rights committed against nurses in this country, against the backdrop of colonialism and apartheid.

LAHLEKILE

The two Statutory Structures, the South African Nursing Association [SANA] and the South African Nursing Council [SANC] grounded their modus operandi in the Nursing Act of 1957. This Act was passed on the premise that discrimination between black and white nurses was appropriate, based on the alleged inferiority of Blacks. Nursing administrators and matrons had testified to this when summoned to Cape Town before the Act was passed. [1:65].

In my personal orbit in the nursing world, we were stunned in 1997 when Mr. Germishuizen, one of the major actors in the SANC, made feather-light testimony before the Truth and Reconciliation Commission. No mention was made of the Human Rights violations of nurses, little apology tabled for unfair labour practices. The true facts will be unearthed in this work.

The alleged inferiority of Blacks has its taproot in Europe. The Victoria Hospital strike in 1949 prompted the late Robert Sobukwe (as quoted) to say:
"The battle is on. To me the struggle at the hospital is more than a question of "discipline". It is a struggle between Africa and Europe, between a twentieth century desire for self-realisation and a feudal conception of authority. The trouble at the hospital then, I say, should be viewed as part of a broad struggle and not as an isolated incident." [1:61]

It is no secret that the state had deliberately set out to suppress the nursing mindset. Nurses had to be "a-political". They were expected to stand as observers to the macro-political transformation of their country from colonialism to apartheid through to democracy. Saccharine ethics as one of the tools used, pontification of the noble role of the nurse, almost to saturation point. No postgraduate student could pass the first year under UNISA** without regurgitating The Eurocentric ethics.

There were structural mechanisms too, which supported the covert belief in "white superiority". These were identified by nurse delegates at a national conference in 1993 [Refer Annexure IV]. It became clear then, that nurses held the key to their liberation in their own hands.

There are no overt signs at the cutting edge of the century that doctors are being re-oriented from the old pattern of male domination. Yet there are ominous indications of black nursing service managers re-writing the old rules of hierarchical oppression. Whether the issue of Human Rights pertaining to nurses is understood is another matter shrouded in mystery. If the current exodus to the Middle East is anything to go by, then a new determination is emerging that nurses will have their economic rights addressed even if this means abandoning their country for foreign soil.

The time has come on this last historical lap for nurses of this country to take their place in history. The respondents of this work spoke openly about the burning issues, which scalded their careers. They bear testimony to the depravity of colonialism and apartheid. Their experiences affirm the magnificent contribution that they were able to make despite having been pointedly ignored by white nurse authors.

There can be no doubt that South Africa *owes* its nurses. May the entire world salute them.
*The term black refers to all ethnic groups not classified as whites.

LAHLEKILE

**University of South Africa.

ACKNOWLEDGEMENT

I wish to express my deep appreciation to the many nurses who were generous enough to share their experiences with me. In doing so, they have validated the political struggle of South African nurses.

A profound word of gratitude to the 'Friends of the Dora Nginza Society' for hosting me when several retirees who had "taken the package" at that time, could be interviewed. These ladies came in strength to provide a major authentic voice for the mid-century trainees.

A special word of appreciation to the countless colleagues throughout the land who provided constant encouragement through the years; most especially Nomaza Majundana, Sanna Joyi, Ella Crisp, Esmé Moses (now late), Aspi Siyola, Mymoena Krysler, Mirriam Rahman, Alice Consul, Glenda Wildschutte, Gail Andrews, and others too numerous to mention.

In the final analysis, the writing of Lahlekile based on nursing testimonies, was therapeutic for me. The anger and frustration of my own life as a professional nurse in *apartheid South Africa* simply fell away and allowed space for personal growth and development.

It is a joy to acknowledge other profoundly special people:

Kiesha Lewis, who tirelessly typed the many drafts with tremendous vitality, a questioning mind and a sense of fun.

LAHLEKILE

Niik Boogchway, who 'fooled around' with my gripe of the 'hand-maiden' role and then came up with the cover design.

Nomsa Tshingila, Kathy Sutton and Euclid Doans for their constant assistance and valuable support. Without them the manuscript might not have materialised.

(Dr) kriben Pillay, who encouraged me to brave the difficulties of getting published.

Shirley Bell, for unstinting editing and the recognition that Lahlekile was an 'important social document' that had to be published.

Christopher Harper, for trying out his photographic skills on me.

Finally, my daughter and son, **Lesley Anne and Roger** respectively, for their endless patience to see my work come to fruition.

ARRANGEMENT OF MATERIAL

The process of selecting material from the first draft was entirely eclectic.

I had to use a guillotine on four hefty manuscripts while colleagues were saying "what you have there is pure gold."

My final decision was to allow the voice of my respondents to come through around specific topics. These could be motivation, training, crisis management or the like.
In this way, I was able to arrange the oral account akin to discussion mode, a methodology that the professional editor-cum-critic – Shirley Bell - was to find captivating.

Important to note then is that the work is designed to highlight the collective experience culminating in the "trends" at the end of the chapter.

It is with profound regret that some contributions had to be left out. None of it will be lost though as the material could be used again in other forms. All respondents are sincerely thanked for their contribution to the whole.

My abiding regret is, that once it was agreed not to disclose the surnames of respondents {with a few exceptions}, I was unable to acknowledge them individually as I'd have liked to do, not having taken down their surnames.
There were two exceptions:

LAHLEKILE

Firstly, Mrs. Ben Mazwi, who became the first black matron. She had gone to England on her own to study theatre technique. As Nanziwe, she tells the story of her subsequent struggle to break the back of apartheid in the operating theatre. Her nursing peers spoke of her with enormous respect, most particularly for the leadership she provided during a time of acute crisis.

Secondly, Miss Gladys Arkel, who was a renowned nursing activist in Cape Town during the period when the profession was dominated by SANA. She became entangled in the dichotomy of either taking up the political struggle from the outside, where a belligerent attitude prevailed, or 'fighting from within.'

When she chose the latter course, she was accosted by angry nurses who appended the term 'stooges' to those who chose to fight from within.

All respondents are most sincerely thanked once again. Without their testimonies this history could not have been captured.

CHAPTER I

PART I - THE FIRST PIONEERS:

CECELIA MAKIWANE

At the turn of the century the only training open to black girls was basic housekeeping. Ward maids were allowed cleaning duties inside hospitals and black girls were popular as domestic servants to urban white housewives in and around Johannesburg.

It was Dr Neil Mac Vicar of Lovedale, who tested the water for nurse training. First he awarded "Leaving Certificates" to his young protégés until he became thoroughly convinced that black inferiority was a social myth.

The Victoria Hospital was his training base. This hospital, together with the Lovedale Institution and Fort Hare University, formed a triangle of educational campuses around the Tyhumie River in Alice, Ciskei (1:58). Neil Mac Vicar knew that he was swimming against the tide but he began to prepare his trainees professionally with great determination.

The very first girl to pass was Miss Cecelia Makiwane, the daughter of a Presbyterian Minister at Mac Farlane Mission about 12km outside Alice. Her passing of the state examination caused an international stir so great that – like Florence Nightingale – she began to ail. It is very likely that she could not understand the fuss or the backdrop against which it was played off.

LAHLEKILE

Miss Makiwane's health began to decline as the pressure took its toll on her apparently frail young body. She was given indefinite sick leave. Her father decided to send her to Johannesburg to the home of Professor Jabavu and his wife, who was her sister. In that house a warm and caring atmosphere was created, close relatives and friends tiptoeing in and out of her room, overcome by her great fame. Unfortunately she never recovered. Death came at a very young age.

Cecelia Makiwane's achievement deserved all the acclaim it got – first registered nurse, first black to pass the state exam. Many years later this was forgotten by the matrons and nurse administrators who avidly testified to black inferiority for the Nursing Act of 1957.

Cecelia's achievement could also be viewed as outstanding against the social background of the rural area. Her great fortune was having a progressive father who valued education. Her eldest sister had become famous too, as the first African woman to have matriculated with mathematics as one of her subjects.

Today Miss Makiwane stands immortalised by:

(1)   A Statue in the hospital grounds where she trained.

(2)   The Cecelia Makiwane Medal of Honour for the "African Nurse of the Year".

(3)   A hospital – Cecelia Makiwane Hospital - was named after her, putting her name on the lips of generations to come (1:52).

Doreen Merle Foster

IN THE AFTERMATH OF CECELIA MAKIWANE'S SUCCESS

To the enquiring contemporary mind a niggling question persists. Why did the simple fact of a young girl passing the state examination become an event that rocked the world off its early century moorings? Could it be that across Europe Blacks were simply not perceived as equal to Whites?

This is very possible judging by the words (as quoted) of Cecil John Rhodes who said, "I contend that we are the finest race in the world and that the more of the world that we inhabit, the better it is for the human race. Just fancy those parts at present inhabited by the most despicable specimens of human beings. What an alteration there would be if they were brought under Anglo-Saxon influence." (2:45).

One great thing that Miss Makiwane's success did was to prove to South Africans and the missionaries from other lands that black inferiority was a concept invented in Europe. She turned a wrong belief on its head. Yet this was not openly admitted. Not a single hospital would accept black nurses for many years to come. In 1916 Miss F.E. Shepherd from England submitted a proposal for midwifery training at the St Monica's Home in Cape Town. The Colonial Medical Council accepted her proposal on the proviso that the courses be presented by a medical doctor. As a consequence Dr Simpson Wells was invited to instruct student midwives.

LAHLEKILE

The trained Nurse's Association opposed the programme, as they did not want a "Coloured" midwife to have the same certificate as a "White". They petitioned the Colonial Medical Council to grant a second-grade certificate to "Coloured" trainees and further stated that she should work under "European" supervision and that her training be extended to two years as compared with the required six months.

However, as reported, "The Medical Council took no notice of these objections" (Reference 3).

TANDIWE JACOBS

Mrs Tandiwe Jacobs was one of the first black nurses ever seen on the streets as a district nurse. She had trained under Dr Mac Vicar too, at the time when they were issued with Leaving Certificates. Her first post was in Cradock where her presence caused a sensation in the African Community.

She was extremely dark; so much so says her daughter (Mrs Ben Mazwi), that there was speculation from the street audience that she was a foreigner from a far distant land. Each time she stepped out of the clinic the people followed her, eyes popping, mouths a-gape.

On a bright summer day she was accosted by a bouncing young lady who fired a barrage of questions at her while standing arms akimbo. Who was she please? What was nursing then? Could she become one too?

Nurse Tandiwe was blessed with a bubbling sense of humour and was amused at the feverish excitement of the pint-sized girl confronting her on her district round.

Willingly she assisted the curious young lady with a draft application and later facilitated her entry into Lovedale. She could not have had any idea that her protégé was to become one of the greatest nurses of the twentieth century.

That young lady, who was so brimful of energy and ambition, turned out to be none other than Dora Nginza. Tandiwe's daughter says: "It is naturally a matter of intense pride in the family that my mother was instrumental in assisting Dora Nginza up the first wrung of the ladder of nursing.

Nurse Tandiwe Jacobs had one or two streets named after her in the Eastern Cape of South Africa. For many years she delivered babies in the Tsolo Location (later to become Duncan Village) of East London. Her portrait hung in the Art Gallery of Fort Hare University and in 1962 she received a TRIBUTE OF COMMENDATION from the Municipality of East London for "loyal and devoted service".

DORA NGINZA 1916

Dora was born to Mr and Mrs Hermanus Jacob Nyamezele on the farm Baviaanspoort near Cradock on 17th October 1891. Her parents were illiterate but their sons Frank and John progressed to the level of trained policemen.

When the sons realised that so-called Coloured policemen earned more money than their black counterparts, they took their father's second name Jacob, added an "s" and got themselves registered as "Coloured" on the police salary sheets.

LAHLEKILE

They had no regrets with this change because the Nginza identity as born and bred Xhosas was virtually cast in stone. It was a time when such matters did not take much weight with the law. Their father died when Dora was a young child so she received her schooling as "Jacobs".

It was a time too when African society firmly believed that girls had to be "fed fat like oxen "(4:1) so that good gains could be had from her labola. Young Dora was contemptuous of this outlook. She struggled against the inbred resistance to education and progress for women.

Circumstances worked in her favour. Her brothers enjoyed salaried employment and gave her a greater measure of freedom than was normally permitted to girls of her age. When she decided to finish her education in the city of Port Elizabeth they gave in, knowing that there was no stopping Dora once an idea had lodged in her brain.

It is assumed that the training years went without a hitch. Neil Mac Vicar was not to know then what deep inroads she would come to make in the lives of thousands of people. It is known that she looked upon the day that she passed her final examination as one of the most important days of her life.

In 1923 a four–year old boy accidentally drank paraffin and was brought to the clinic. Sister Dora without hesitation performed a medical procedure – a stomach washout – for which she was hailed, having snatched the child from the jaws of death. A few years later the same child fell off a donkey and Sister Dora attended to his fractured arm.

This was the beginning of a life-long relationship. As a child in the 1930's the growing boy spent his afternoons at the clinic as a volunteer for odd jobs. As a young man he became a junior clerk under Sister Dora. Eventually, he departed for tertiary education in England where he qualified as a librarian.

He was Mr G Soya Mama who became a noted writer and poet. In the book "Indyebo Ka-Xhosa" he published six of his poems in an anthology, along with six other poets' work. This anthology is regarded as a treasure in Xhosa literature. It is used in lectures at the University of South Africa by the Department of African languages. One of the poems by Mr Mama is a song he was commissioned to write when community leaders wished to commemorate Sister Dora's birthday in 1951. (5:3)

Her husband was Chief Hendry Nginza. They lived with their adopted son and daughter in the "White Location" in New Brighton, Port Elizabeth. It is not known whether she had a problem of infertility but the children they adopted were both blood relatives of the Nginza family.

The son Velile Nginza was nicknamed "Countryman". He was much older than Christine the daughter. He became addicted to alcohol and died of alcohol abuse. When Christine gave testimony to her mother's life many years later, she recalled their upbringing.

"Countryman and I were raised with great love. Any child raised by a mother such as her and somehow loses his way, cannot look to lay the blame at her door. She had made me what I am today – up to the haste in me –

for when she gave you a task to do it had to be done at once. And you had to listen carefully to what she said. There was no turning back to ask, "What is it that you want done Mama?" You had to be very alert, that is what she taught me."

Sister Dora had strong leadership qualities with a measure of dominance. She was seen as brisk and efficient. Throughout the Eastern Cape she became known and respected, a much admired figure to girls of all ages.

One of these was a little girl called Chrissie whose home was situated near the clinic. One can imagine a quick cup of tea during brief moments snatched from her busy days. Chrissie too gave testimony to Sister Dora's life. She did this at the age of 70 years as Mrs Harmans.

"As a young girl I was overwhelmed by her. Not only the uniform but by witnessing her efficiency. I decided that I would follow in the great nurse's footsteps when I grew up."

Mrs Harmans then related how hard she and her peers had to work from 1941 onwards. Her dream had come true when she secured a post under Sister Dora. However the reality was harsh. For one thing the salary was so paltry that she would not bother to recall directly how much it had been; for another they had to deliver a comprehensive service. It was no easy ride.

Frequently Sister Dora took up the mantle of teacher, lecturing on aspects of practice. She was fluent in Xhosa, English, Afrikaans and South-Sotho. She carried the titles MOTHER OF NEW BRIGHTON and MOTHER

OF THE NATION because she was living proof to the tethered women of the time that it was possible for a woman to attain her fullest potential.

A! NOBANTU (Mother of the Nation) is the very highest respect that could befall a woman. With her distinctive limp she bore the title with dignity.

The limp had begun in the early 40's when she had rushed to assist her husband when he had collapsed nears the gates of the house one fateful day.

Headman John Henry Ginza was a caretaker at the T.C. White Recreational Hall within a stone's throw of their house. One day he was about to set out for work when his body packed up without warning. His wife found him crumpled up on the ground.

Without hesitation she picked him up bodily and carried him inside. Although she was a strong woman she suffered a hip injury which surgery (at that time) could not correct. Consequently she remained handicapped by the limp.

Her husband died on 12th September 1943. His death caused a marked deficit – not only in her personal life and in the home – but also within the tribe. A new headman had to be found. Usually the deceased headman had to be replaced by his son but due to Countryman's addiction to alcohol, this was not possible.

In 1945 the supreme chief of the Ama-Rarabe (pronounced Ama-Gaggabie): Archibald Velile Sandile, bestowed the chieftainship on her. Until her death she remained the representative of the Eastern Cape Urban

Area, conferring and deliberating with males on civic matters. These males were Xhosa representatives; she led her own delegation in council sittings where she was able generally to play a leadership role.

Meanwhile she not only carried out civic and professional duties but gave of her abundant energy to the church too, both as devoted member and as Sunday school teacher. Her achievements go far beyond the magnificent and are almost too numerous to mention. In 1991 a tribute to her appeared in the Weekend Post [ref. 6] from which her principle achievements can be summarised:

1. She was amongst the first batch of black nurses [soon after Cecelia Makiwane's first-ever group of three] who trained at the Lovedale Mission Hospital under Dr Neil Mac Vicar.

2. Appointed by the Government as the first health visitor of New Brighton.

3. Commended for her early recognition of typhoid fever during an epidemic, which occurred six months after she took up her post.

4. In 1925 she received the Prince of Wales at the clinic where (as quoted in 5) imbongi Samuel Edward Krune Mqhayi, known as the "Father of Xhosa poetry" sang the Prince's praises.

5. In 1927 she went to Switzerland and England as a member of the Moral Re-Armament Movement.

6. Received a presentation in 1951 from the New York Council of African Affairs – the first black woman to receive the award made annually to those who had done work of public benefit among people in Africa.

7. The hall of the Newell Congregational Church was named after her, the A! Nobantu Hall.

8. She was presented with a Xhosa bible with the following inscription: *IN DEEP APPRECIATION OF THE UNSELFISH service rendered on the occasion of the 8th Bantu Convention in Port Elizabeth 18-21 December, 1945.*

9. Paramount Chief Sandile presented her with an illuminated address in 1954 upon her retirement.

10. She was commended by the (former) M.O.H. Dr J.N. Sher as "An outstanding personality, highly respected; she was fluent in English and Afrikaans and kept company with the V.I.P.'s of those days."

11. An NGO has been established in her name, the "Friends of the Dora Nginza society."

12. Upon her retirement she was presented with a blanket by SANA.

In conclusion it must be noted that on a cold, windy day when Dr A.T. Van Wyk [retired lecturer in history at UNISA] was received by Mrs Orlayne [current chief nursing service manager] and her staff for the purpose of capturing Dora Nginza's history, the superintendent *

LAHLEKILE

[Dr Waynratty] was apparently overwhelmed by the information put on the table that day in 1987.

He subsequently wrote in a hospital publication: "Let us strive to become what already is being said about us, that Dora Nginza's spirit has taken hold of the personnel.
In fact, I now realise why this hospital has been named after her."

Dora Nginza became a legendary figure in her time. The hospital is a living monument to one of the greatest women of the 20th century.

Reference 5, 7, 11

* Editor not certain that the superintendent's name was correctly recorded. Taken from a rather old notebook.

THE UNSUNG PIONEERS

CONTRIBUTORS TO THIS SECTION:

1. **Zoë**
2. **Johanna**
3. **Evelina**
4. **Cornelia**
5. **Nomsa**

PRELUDE

On a dusty sun-baked road in South West Africa (now Namibia) a merry crowd of low-income workers trudged along in a spirit of abandonment. They were on their way to a wedding, a rare event in their drab lives.

Zoë's throat felt as dry as the red earth around them. The African heat made the thought of a glass of cold water prick at her salivary glands. The wedding venue was miles away and already her feet were sore in the new leather sandals that bound them.

She was barely twenty-three years old. The people called her "sister", this tall girl with blue eyes set in sharp features, blonde frizzy hair kept short, an attractive hybrid from South Africa's Transkei region. The crowd moved with boundless energy. Zoë suspected that the men were secretly sipping from a hidden bottle. Already their dominant Khoi features were flattened in laughter at their own cracking wit. Old Jonas had deep crows feet under his eyes and Attie's face looked like a road map.

LAHLEKILE

Young Abraham was blowing a mouth organ, showing rotten teeth and much saliva in the process.

The women strode proudly behind the men, buttocks jouncing, heads wrapped in brilliantly coloured "doeks". Their garish gayety added a touch of barbaric splendour to the outing. Zoe was proud to be a central figure in their lives for her work was all she lived for.

"Look sister, there's Jimmy". Zoë was jerked back to the present by Attie's excited voice. And true enough there was a familiar truck brought to a screeching halt. The driver had been requested by the magistrate to provide motor transportation for Zoe whenever he visited the locations. He was an Indian businessman who sold firewood and happily took the young nurse along but this arrangement was not acceptable to the wife who became hysterical over the issue more often than not.

"Going to the wedding?" called Jimmy the driver, "Well, hop on everyone, we're going too." Suddenly the wife poked her head through the window and screamed, "No, no, not her - she's not coming with us." Attie put his arm protectively around Zoë. With a clown's gift for comedy he said, "Come along Sister, don't worry your pretty little head about her." He promptly scooped her up in his arms and positioned her at the back of the truck. Then he took the stance of a traffic officer to get everyone on board.

With boisterous laughter and song they were off, unrestrained voices shattering the morning peace. With skins glistening in the African heat they proceeded to the wedding in great merriment.

The year was 1930 and the wedding was one of a few social events that Zoë was able to dredge from memory 70 years later. It seems that her life was so crammed with professional duties that she had no time left for the experiences of marriage and motherhood. Her entire productive life was given to nursing.

THE SMILES AND TEARS OF OUR WORKING YEARS

ZOË

I was orphaned at an early age and grew up in Kokstad in the Transkei under an aunt who was the only relative I had. My training began in 1925 at the Lovedale Missionary Institution. At that time we were first given a Leaving Certificate until Dr Neil Mac Vicar found us ready to try the Colonial Medical Council exam.

We were not allowed to sit at Frere Hospital East London because only white nurses were allowed to write there. Dr Mac Vicar arranged for us to write at the Port Elizabeth Provincial Hospital. He said, "You must do well because I'm fighting for you girls to have the same certificate and the Europeans don't want that."

There was discrimination with patients too. I once had to attend to the grandchild of an elderly Afrikaner woman when I was a clinic nurse in South West Africa. The health inspector requested that I attend to that child. Naturally I was curious so I asked why they were not going to the hospital. To my astonishment she replied,

"Hulle wil nie vir ons help nie want ons is arm." (They do not want to help us because we are poor).

At a later stage the same old lady took ill and earnestly came knocking at my door. This time the health inspector would not allow me to take care of her so he thought of a plan. I was to accompany her to the hospital saying that we were only taking her in for tests. In the car she clung to me, sobbing bitterly. She said that she dreaded falling into the hands of the white nurses. Our journey up the steps of the hospital was slow and to this day I cannot forget the tearful blaming look she gave me over her shoulder as they led their reluctant patient inside.

JOHANNA

My training began as a lark. Long before formal training I learned how to deliver babies from two white nurses. I was working as a domestic servant in the Nurses' Home in Graaf Reinet when they befriended me. They said, "You're not meant for bed making and to be a tea girl." Once I learned how to deliver babies they were happy to leave me to it when their boyfriends came to visit.

The biggest problem at the start of my career as a midwife was my mother. Her strict Victorian values would not allow me to find out where babies came from. This made me very curious but before my stay in Graaf Reinet it was impossible for me to get a peek through the secret door. Maybe they thought that children would fall into a black hole or something if they found out where babies come from. It was only when I took to my bed with flue that Mother found out which way the wind was blowing. The nurses rushed to the house "You can't lie in bed Johanna, your babies need you." Mother dropped something and her eyes grew big as saucers. "What does she know about babies?" So they told her "Your little girl is far from innocent. She is a *nurse*."

At the insistence of my aunt who was her self a professional nurse I registered for training in Port Elizabeth but halfway through I dropped out. I had so much practical experience by then that I just did not feel like studying all the stuff they put before you. All those sisters who trained me are dead now anyway.

I was allowed to open my own practice under the Walmer Municipality in Port Elizabeth using the clinic as my base. The Clinic authorities regularly inspected my uniform – a white dress worn by all nurses – my bag and my register. I took pride in my appearance and kept my equipment in order. Everything was very clean otherwise you risked being sacked. I bought all my own things – cotton wool, thermometer, Dettol, spirits, eye-drops.

Throughout my thirty years of practice I worked very hard but not for riches. Sometimes the people had no money to pay me. If I got to a poor house I often had to dip into my own pocket to give what I could. At other times I only took bus fare. If they could pay the fees, that was okay but mostly I worked without pay because my husband looked after me, so I was independent in work.

My poor income worried the other nurses. "How much do you charge?" They wanted to know but I kept my lips sealed because that was my business, I thought. One day Nurse Meyer (my Aunt) took me aside in her car. "You must stop working for nothing, you must make the people pay," she said crossly. We argued about it. I said, "You've got lots of money Auntie, those people have nothing. The babies must have clothes and nappies, why must I still take from them?

My best friend in work was Dr Appavoo. I never called upon him or any other doctor for help and I'm proud of that, but he often came to visit me at home and liked to give his cases to me for delivery. Sometimes, Dr Appavoo was so surprised at me. He would say, "How did you do that?" I would shrug and say "Ag, he just walked out doctor." My feeling was that I was not alone, that God guided these two hands to do the work. (She held up hands brown as cinnamon, adorned with a plain wedding band.)

I had some very difficult cases at times. One was the delivery of my own granddaughter. On the night of the delivery my daughter-in-law became restless and fretful. "Why is it taking so long?" She cried. Her first experience had been smooth as a knife going through butter but now she was having trouble and getting hysterical too. "Why is it so funny this time?" she whined. I said firmly, "Just keep your mouth shut. I don't need man here I need God."

The baby's bum was at the face of the birth canal and the two legs were around the head from behind. It was a struggle to bring those legs down. I bring one down over the head and start with the other, but the first would jump back again. Soon I asked the Lord for help. After that it wasn't ten minutes and the legs were down. I then brought her out sideways (graphic hand gestures) with the head and then the arms. That's how my granddaughter was born.

I had many difficult cases, too many, but never once did my patients suffer a tear. They trusted me when I said; "don't push now" and that saved them from tears. Even when their doctors sent them to the hospital to give birth they would come to me first, lie on the bed and ask that I palpate them just to see that everything was alright. Another difficulty I had was going out at night to deliver white babies. Some husbands would try to make a pass at me but I remained poker-faced. They then left me alone.

I had a work companion, an African nurse. Those days there was no discrimination especially not between African and "Coloured" people. We worked nicely together. Whenever she had problems in delivery she would come to me.

One busy day this happened again. My area stretched around South End, Fairview Mount, Salisbury Park, Mount Pleasant as well as the surrounding farms. I did those areas mostly on foot in all weathers, sometimes by bus. On that day I was extremely tired and decided to go home for a short rest, only to find my children very excited. Nurse Majoka had been there and needed to see me urgently, they said.

Hardly was I able to take a few sips of tea when she came through the door like a whirlwind. "Oh man, you've got to help me today. The baby was born 5 o'clock this morning and I can't get the placenta out." "Why didn't you phone a doctor to come and help you?" She ignored the irritability in my voice and said "Oh no, I first want you to come and see."

LAHLEKILE

Off we went. I got that placenta out in two ticks. Look, I don't mean to brag but God gave me this gift to bring babies safely into the world. My husband helped me a lot by building a big house for me in Stanford Road. Even after retirement I still sit on the step each day with a cup of coffee to watch the first bus go by.

I retired in 1970 after a car accident left me with an injured leg. The nurses came running to ask me to work for a few more years but my heart was heavy too. Not only did my husband pass on but also the Municipality said I could only deliver "Coloured" babies. To my mind God didn't have any colour and babies were the same but they had other ideas all of a sudden. It made my heart very sore.

Anyway, I went to the Livingstone Hospital a while ago (1990) to visit a friend who was sick. While there I heard a patient next door call "Nurse, Nurse!" Putting my head outside the door I saw a young nurse and an Indian doctor standing very close. They were flirting and did not hear the patient call.

My friend saw me getting up and said, "Don't go in there Johanna, the nurses can be rude if you interfere." But I pushed open the door and entered. There was the patient falling out of her cushions and bearing down.

At once I used my fingers to check and located the baby's head. My fear was that should the water break – for it was yet to do so – then that plastic will go down with the baby. You have to jump in otherwise the baby will die; he or she will drown in the water.

It was a little boy that I delivered that day, twenty years after retirement. I lifted him up to clear the air passage then lay him down nicely on the bed before I rang the bell.

"Who rings the bell?" asked a nurse in a fighting manner. I said, "It's me. I ring the bell. Come and pay attention to your work."

So they came at last, only to find the baby delivered. If he had drowned face down in the bag of waters they would just have written <u>still born</u>. But he was alive. I saved him.

EVELINA

I commenced training in 1936 in the heart of Zululand at St Mary's hospital, which was situated at a place called Ntenemeda at Quamadada. It was an Anglican mission with a church just a short distance away.

I went into training in a delirium of expectation because during my study years (Junior Certificate in Bloemfontein) I had helped a district nurse on a voluntary basis during a typhus epidemic. We took blankets and sheets into a special room where the lice were chemically destroyed.

During the training period we had to do everything – washing, cooking for patients and all the cleaning jobs too. It was extremely hard work but we maintained a dignified exterior. Being young, elation danced within.

Miss Balmain, a kind lady from Scotland, was our matron and tutor. She was assisted by Sister Lizzie Allen. Our doctor was Dr Bandow who used to travel once a week to the very heart of Zululand. This was on-the-job training with classes three times a week. I loved it all. Matron was tough as teak, ready to gobble up anyone who erred but she and Sister Lizzie both earned our boundless admiration and trust.

The morning bell rang at 5am for us to get up, get dressed and off to chapel and prayers. This was followed by breakfast. We had a rotation system where we spent 3 months in a ward, 3 in the kitchen and 3 months in the laundry. In the process of work we were straining our young backs. At night we used lanterns; electricity was reserved for the theatre.

CORNELIA

I was born in Paarl (about 70km out of Cape Town) where I attended school at the Zion Primary, an offshoot of the Dutch Reformed Church.

In 1939 I undertook midwifery at St Monica's in Cape Town. Our matron was Miss Hefford from England. St Monica's was an Anglican mission hospital under Bishop Lavis. We who were Dutch Reformed worshippers had to attend church on the mornings when he officiated. An excited murmur would rip through the ranks – "Bishop is coming!" I felt like a frightened child in a maze for to me, everything in the Anglican form of worship was very foreign.

We aliens would not partake in communion of course, but we were compelled to attend the services so we sang the hymns and joined in the prayers. After the service we'd all sit around the huge dining room table to have breakfast with the Bishop of Cape Town.

Our tutors were Sister Thomas and Dr Simpson–Wells. He always had the junior nurses sitting at the back of the class, the senior's under his nose. To them it was that he directed all his questions so that left us juniors plenty of time to skylark.

Our uniforms consisted of stiff collars and celluloid cuffs. These we wore with blue dresses covered by white aprons. We wore broad belts, thick black stockings and black shoes. The cap was folded from a huge triangular cloth. We were given the dictum, *"the cap is there to protect your hair."*

Every Friday we were fed dry beans. During Lent this became a form of torture for then we had dry beans on Tuesdays too. Other days we were given mealie-meal pap or kaffir corn, but the golden rule was beans on Fridays.

I was given the task of going to the laboratory on Friday mornings. I would quietly scrape the beans into my handkerchief and get rid of it one at a time all the way to the lab. Sister Thomas would time and again inspect the dirt bin, her face distorted like a lemon. Her mission was to discover who had wasted "the wholesome food that God provides." Often she would report to Miss Hefford about whole boiled potatoes lying in the bin.

NOMSA

My first name Lydia is a white name and I'm not going to use that name because I am not white. My motivation for nursing came from seeing a nurse while I was at home. She was a Miss Machaka who was smart, clean, attractive and very trim. I so admired her athletic figure when she played tennis. She was so very beautiful that I decided to become a nurse too.

I began training at the King Edward Hospital in Durban (1940) but at the official opening of the hospital we learned that Africans would receive only a "Hospital Certificate" while the five "Indian" students (born and bred in South Africa) would become registered nurses. All of us had matriculated and most of them had only Junior Certificates. Of course this discrimination was unacceptable and we had no hesitation in leaving.

I went to the nearest place that offered proper training, the Holy Cross. There was a connection between the Anglican Holy Cross and the Mc Cord Hospital which was an American missionary hospital situated in Durban. They had a working arrangement for us to proceed with midwifery after general and this suited us to the ground.

The training years were most enjoyable, the missionaries so very nice. What the students simply loved was the compulsory church attendance. Those who were day-off were excused but first their names had to be written on a slate. On the Sunday when you were off, the duty nurses went to church and your turn would be on the following Sunday. The duty nurses loved being in church during duty hours.

We were terribly pampered at the mission hospitals. The maids brought breakfast to us on trays while we were still in bed. It gave us a sense of human worth. We were also allowed to play tennis and have parties. The late Oliver Tambo was one of our boyfriends. Those were lovely days, the most memorable and the most enjoyable. All the staff at Holy Cross were from overseas.

<u>EVELINA</u>

We enjoyed our training years despite the hardships. We were young, naughty and full of expectations. The hospital was surrounded by a small forest where the air was drenched with the scent of wild flowers. Behind the chapel we had a garden, which gave us access to fruit fresh from its trees. This was a succulent supplement to a really awful diet served up to the student nurses.

Most of our meals consisted of mealies or "madumbe" which was nothing more than porridge and milk. We had to eat what the local people ate, something I could not understand the logic of.

Our baker was a very kind man. He crossed my horizon because he discovered my name and said that his wife's name was "Evelina" too. Whenever he saw my tearful face he would say, "Don't cry, I shall make a special loaf for you. His Zulu was like a beautiful song. He would say, "Come Evelina, come little one, don't cry. We shall teach you to speak Zulu."

Each day we fell about our chores washing patients, feeding them, doing their pressure parts. And observing. At that time there was no technology, no antibiotics, so we had to watch the patients very closely, especially the pneumonia suffers. They would lie there and cry "Nurse, Nurse!"

We moved through the days in a mighty restrained rhythm. It was so cold in winter that you felt it penetrate to your very bones. Great care was given to the washing of hands for which a bowl of carbolic water was kept nearby. It was very basic those days but it was a good learning experience.

I remember a little girl of about 14 years of age who was brought in from one of the kraals. She was hollowed out by starvation, all crimped up with feet and legs turned inwards. Her bone-thin body had bloated lice crawling all over it. You could see how she clenched her teeth each time the vermin bit and her pitiful attempts to scratch.

We students began to froth around the newcomer. On the one hand there was the abandonment of this child by her family. On the other there were the apostles of mercy who had brought her in. They exuded a conviction that somehow the hospital would see the situation right. We felt the tension. It ran like a crack in the earth's crust.

Our first reaction was to flee from the absolute horror of it all, but Sister Lizzie's voice pounded out a warning: "No, no, no. It is not for us to be judgmental. Our task is to relieve her stress. She then proceeded to direct us in the task of cleansing. I saw her pour something in the bath water but cannot remember what it was, only that it was not Dettol.

We had to use cotton-wool rather than a cloth and we dabbed carefully for the skin was coming off, having shrivelled in the tropical sun. Sister Lizzie took a large bottle of cod-liver oil in which she soaked strips of lint, which she then used to cover the entire body area. It was an enormous yet delicate task.

The patient's mouth was so stiff we could not get any food past her clenched teeth. She seemed to be in a state of mysterious stupor. It was Sister Lizzie who was able to get some nourishing fluid through.

She was given the name "Lathegile" by the people who had brought her in. It means "thrown away." Lathegile managed to live for a few days. Under our ministrations she had grimly hung on to the last shreds of life.

<u>ZOË</u>

I had a difficult time with an Indian Businessman's wife. The magistrate of Windhoek had requested that whenever he sold firewood to people in the locations, that he transports me as an accredited passenger of the state. Often he obligingly brought patients through by car.

This arrangement caused endless problems with the man's wife. Whenever she spotted me she would throw a jealous tantrum at any public point. Once she knocked on my door at home. I opened it to find her standing on the doorstep like an angry Nefertiti. She held out slender arms dripping with jewellery but sporting red wheels as well. "Jimmy het my geslaan" was all that she could say. (Jimmy has beaten me).

On another occasion she came to the clinic where she poured verbal abuse on my head in front of the patients. The people were angry, called a taxi and bundled me into it with several others. "Come on sister, we'll put a stop to this nonsense."

At the courthouse the magistrate sat with an enamelled mask of correctness listening to the story and then asking me questions. Finally he told me to return to the clinic and continue with my work. Then he sent for the husband to tell him to keep his wife in check. I remember getting through the rest of that day in a mild shock of anti-climax.

CORNELIA

The St Monica's Home was in Bree Street Cape Town while our residential quarters was in Buitengracht Street. On Saturdays we were given clean bed linen. It was a chance for Matron to scold us for wrongdoing; any misdemeanours that she happened to have chalked up against any person. We stood at attention in long rows like recruits in the Army. She would turn from one to the other as if she were a wire.

One day I had come from the labour ward to the lying-in ward. I had no idea what was happening but I came just at the time when Dr Simpson-Wells was informing Matron that one of the patient's intake and output had not been charted. When questioned about the oversight the ward nurse stated that I was the culprit, a lie, which truly appalled me.

Well, the very next Saturday Miss Hefford gave me hell. "You come here with marvellous testimonials but you're not worth the paper it's written on" she ranted. I spent the rest of that Saturday drenched in tears.

There was an older nurse from Wellington who was in fact already a grandmother. She became very disgruntled when Matron's scolding had cast its shadow over her. I found her packing, ready to leave. Hastily I intervened. "You can't do that man; you're already at the end of your course." She opened her mouth and shut it again without saying anything; eyes as darkly purple as plums in chocolate. She was so very angry but I persuaded her to stay.

My first post was in Great Brak River from where I was transferred to Paarl. While there, an inspectress arrived from Pretoria accompanied by a young nurse who became very excited over the Moslem culture she encountered in my district. So much so that she expressed a sudden desire to work amongst the people of Islam.

She seemed overawed by their fussiness with colour. They would deck out the bedroom in lilac one day - curtains, bedding, baby and all - tomorrow it will be pink, the next day lemon. It would be the midwife's fate to assist with the change of linen.

Invariably on the 7th day their male babies would be circumcised. There was also the practice of the flower from Mecca used to predict the opening of the cervix. When that happened the flower would open at the same time. A dry flower like a piece of wood, cinnamon in colour. This flower would be placed in bowl of water, later the water drunk. That is something to see and remember forever.

They also delighted in serving tea to the nurses. This would include spicy biscuits and other delicacies. It was a custom that finally bowled over the young nurse accompanying the inspectress.

LAHLEKILE

Soon after this, just when I returned from my annual leave, I was informed via the grapevine that I was to be moved to the back areas of Paarl while that nurse would take over my district. I felt steamed up by this duplicity and used the power of the pen to write a letter of resignation driven by a sense of outrage. My peaked handwriting spoke to the authorities in no uncertain terms. "Sir, duties under your Board will end on 31st May 1943. Hoping my resignation will be accepted."

My superiors received the letter like a bolt out of the blue. Dr Jager was the chairman of the Board and he promptly sent for me. He pretended a cheerful attitude. "Well, you wrote a resignation but here, write another letter stating "Sir, I wish to withdraw ......"" His tone sounded bossy, the sentence drumming back in my ears.

With bright open eyes I said, "I'm not prepared to be turned out of my area by a stranger. And I won't become a boarder in a town where I own my own home." The fact is that the back areas were so far out it could have been the hinterland.

Peace returned when I was allowed to stay. The supervisor of our districts explained to the avid young lady, "We cannot transfer her because she gave valid reasons to the Board why she should stay." So I clung to my post like a limpet to the side of a mountain.

NOMSA

I once had a patient at the Livingstone Hospital in Port Elizabeth who was bleeding so much, it was as though a water pipe had burst. I flew into a panic and called the doctor. This was an "Indian" doctor whose name I cannot remember but he was later to be arrested and detained for political activism.

The crisis on hand put me in a sweat. While I exuded panic, this doctor remained cool as a cucumber. He worked so beautifully, so calmly and afterwards he lectured me with the patience of a saint. "When you see a patient bleeding like this, don't panic because when you panic you battle to find the veins. You might even cause the veins to collapse and then you won't be able to get the needle in. Do not panic because eventually you are going to give the patient the blood. It's not the hurry which will save the patient, it's the blood."

I learned a lesson from the doctor that day which I shall never forget. I learned from him not to panic, not even when I'm driving and it looks as though something might happen. You can't possibly do anything right if you fly into a flap. If something is bound to happen, then it will. That I believe.

The difficulties of nursing revolved around white attitudes where white and black worked together. There was this unfair arrangement at the Frere Maternity Hospital that when the white sister-in-charge was off from night duty, that she was replaced by one who was very junior to me. I felt that this was an insult. I was far older than her, far more qualified and just because I was black I had to work under her. She used to sleep through most of the night and then erupt on us with assumed white authority the next morning.

I was unpopular at that hospital even with some of the doctors. I resisted their oppression. It was as though we had a canopy over us that was pushing us down. There was a feeling that nothing could ever change for us; the white nurses had it all. As an individual you couldn't change jobs because there were simply no other options so you laboured on without joy, like an ox pulling a plough.

Dr L. especially disliked me because I came across as cheeky to him. One day he stormed at me because a patient was not ready for him. I said, "The patient will be made ready now doctor. I cannot place her in the lithotomic position (legs up in stirrups) when you are not here.

My motivation was that this position was most painful to many women. They could actually be crippled for a long while afterwards if a nerve got pinched. What I did to get around this problem was to divide the bed into two halves. We let the patient lie on one half while on the other we had the poles and everything ready to position her when the doctor came. It was easy to do this in the time it took him to scrub.

As it was, a catastrophe occurred while I was off duty one day. My niece was on and she obediently placed the patient in stirrups before the doctor arrived. While he was scrubbing, the woman suddenly gave a mighty push, expelling the baby at jet force on to the floor. The cord snapped and the baby's life was rudely snuffed out.

The case went to court. My niece had to explain how it happened and the doctor had to tell his side. In fairness to Dr L. he took the blame but (sigh) you know how the whites look after one another, nothing came of the case.

CORNELIA

I once provided service to a very wealthy Muslim family – the Latief family – who lived in an enormous mansion. When the young wives fell pregnant they would not attend the clinic, something that rubbed me up the wrong way. Before my involvement with the case in hand, the young wife had suffered a serious car injury. The doctors had almost given up but she survived to book in with me a year later.

At first I was reluctant to take the case because of their aversion to attending the clinic but the relatives maintained such high spirits, giving me disjointed news whenever they saw me, as to her progress that I accepted the challenge.

According to their observations, "her feet are not swollen yet" so she was obstetrically safe. I found their comments worrying and amusing at the same time. When the first labour pain came on, I was called. There was a sense of something pending that was so tremendous that it gave rise to a fever of excitement.

In the meantime I had to while away hours and hours. I saw the family being cast in a spell, sharing with one another an ecstasy of anticipation. Meanwhile I began to crave for a hot, foamy bath. The family lost all sense of time. They brought me trays loaded with food at such frequent intervals that it was impossible for me to consume most of it.

Finally, when the baby's first cry was heard, their high-pitched tone of hysteria was released on the air. Some were running to the phone, telling people in Cape Town, "We don't know what it is but we hear the baby crying."

NOMSA

In Kimberley we used to go to the patient's homes to deliver their babies. Ours was a comprehensive service. We were only two nurses and we worked around the clock. The distances from one location to another had to be done on foot and after night deliveries you still had to do day duty at the clinic.

The long hours and hard work encroached on your personal life. Often there was no time and energy left for your husband. I got to hate the footsteps coming to the door (laughs uproariously) you might be busy making a cup of tea, hoping to enjoy this in the company of your husband and then the footsteps come, plop-plop-plop.

You would walk out in all weathers. Another thing, which got to you, was the vast poverty. It is simply indescribable. Some people have such a little to get by on and then there are those who have nothing at all. You even have to go next-door to ask for hot water.

When approaching the house for a delivery there's no problem about finding the place even at night because there would always be a curious crowd hovering around. It was not unusual for them to deliver the baby themselves except for cutting of the cord. They somehow knew that would have got them into hot water. When you asked, "who delivered this baby?" they would close ranks and claim that the delivery was spontaneous. The mother would go along with this untruth knowing full well that the "gamp" who delivered the baby would be outside, innocently melted into the crowd.

As soon as everything seemed under control they would slink into the house to ask after the sex of the baby and the health of the mother. (Nomsa's eyes cloud with tears of mirth). They definitely know the sex of the baby but they pretend delight and surprise when told.

ZOË

I once had to nurse a community single-handedly through a typhoid epidemic. That was at Malthoé, which lies en route to the Namib Desert. No one else wanted to volunteer; no one showed any inclination to co-operate with the authorities. My own excuse was my midwifery caseload but there were eager offers of help on that score so that I could not really refuse to go.

I left the Windhoek station at 7:30pm, travelled all night and reached my destination on the following morning. During the journey I saw many beautiful farms before darkness fell, luscious German-owned farms. The next morning I was met at the station by the doctor's "boy" who had, been instructed to take me to the Red Cross sisters until the doctor was able to see me.

At Malthoe I moved all the sick people to the Methodist Church hall. I was given the help of two hospital assistants for soon the place was jammed to capacity around the sides and centre too. I got the women to boil big pots of water at night, which we dispensed into containers in the morning so that the patients had plenty of clean water to drink.

LAHLEKILE

There was no prescribed medicine for typhoid. Before my departure the superintendent of the Windhoek Hospital had unlocked his stores and I was allowed to pack in whatever I thought was necessary. I took plenty of aspirin, also quinine. Penicillin was still very scarce. The assistants did bedpan rounds and attended to the hygiene of the patients. I sponged down frequently those with high temperatures.

The doctor came every two weeks. His car would be spotted in the distance stirring up dust. The people would say, "There goes the doctor, first to the hotel to quench his thirst." After a while he would stroll in full of cheer and say, "Ah, my very good nurse, I know that everything is fine in your hands."

The epidemic petered out after six weeks. All that time I was housed by a Bushman teacher with my food sent three times a day by the hotel and my laundry done by hotel staff.

There were no setbacks to my career except a big disappointment upon retirement. I wrote to my professional body, the SANA, who wrote back that there was nothing that they could do for me. I should apply to the "Coloured Affairs Department" for an old-age pension. They asked though that I send money for their Trust Fund but I didn't. That Trust Fund was for the upkeep of retired white nurses in beautiful homes. I get a pension now and the oddest thing is that it's more money than I ever got when I was working.

EVELINA

Going back to general nursing practice I worked in the university clinic at Alexandria township in 1940 just one year after the war. The situation provided a sobering reminder of realities outside the clinic walls.

We used bicycles as a mode of transport and our little bags contained bandages, aspirin and sulphadiazide. There was not much Penicillin as yet. If it happened that you did not have a bicycle you had to foot it, going from door to door. That was hard work but we were still young.

One interesting happening is indelibly written on my mind. It is the picture I have of Sister Coles who – like Paula of ancient times – went out on case-finding. On the streets she encountered a man lying with his throat cut.

She brought the patient back with her. Around his throat and neck she had put a bandage, which was oozing blood. Sister Coles moved as though in daze. As I looked down at the man whose life was ebbing away, a prickly sensation passed through me. It was utterly appalling. Could it have been a case of "African revenge?" Subtle, cunning beyond revenge exacted anywhere else in the world other than in Mafia circles. I cannot erase that case from my memory.

Nursing definitely needs to change. It has become cold and scientific. There is a preposterous illusion that science is everything, yet the essence of nursing is The Touch. Nursing is in fact a calling.

Of course one has to acknowledge advancement, yet at the same time to realise that the focus on technology has sent patient care for a loop. Let us stay with technology but let's return to love and etiquette, which prevailed before.

Take "middle" for instance. We had no technology with which to detect the foetal heart; all we had were our ears. These days we read in the newspapers about a miraculous operation performed on a foetus while in the uterus. That is excellent, really marvellous. But let's not forget the basics, especially the caring aspect.

NOMSA CONTINUES

The difficulties of nursing revolve around white attitudes one had to endure at a hospital like Frere in East London. There was no upward mobility for me.

I was regarded as a troublemaker because I could articulate my feelings and that affected my chances. Though nurses were allowed to work in the office at times, one matron actually left instructions before she went on leave, that under no circumstances was I to be allowed to work in the office.

A colleague carried the news to me with some glee. I was influencing the other staff members, the matron had said. I replied, "Well, that is an honour for me, if you are telling me that the others have no minds of their own and can be led by me. I don't want their office, thank you very much; I don't need their office at all."

There were no gender problems as such. We worked with white doctors who never treated us as "ladies" as they did the white nurses. It seemed that we blacks were merely their chattels to carry out the necessary work. It was very different at Livingstone where the Indian and black doctors saw us as human beings.

I had problems with doctors but it had nothing to do with gender and everything to do with the colour of my skin. They wanted a master-servant relationship and there was no way that I could give them that.

At another time Doctor S. Came into the labour ward and wanted it cleared of patients immediately. He had no regard for the fact that all the patients were fresh deliveries still in pain or great discomfort. "Out!" he said, "To Ground Floor or to Admissions." I said, "Doctor, I shan't do that. I'll phone the Ground floor ward and ask if there are any beds and if there are none then I shan't sent the patients to Admissions."

His voice became threatening. When he said, "Sister, I want this ward cleared!" I replied, "I'm not sending them to Admissions." He went to the matron and I was called but stood firm. I said, "Nobody sends patients to Admissions for lying in. If I can't get beds in the ward I shall keep them in the labour ward. How are the nurses going to swab patients who are lying on the floor? How can they take blood pressures? How can 24 patients be accommodated on six mattresses on the floor? Even if you send me to the superintendent, I don't care, but the patients will remain in the labour ward.

LAHLEKILE

The next day I was off duty. In my absence that doctor saw to it that his orders were carried out. When I returned, the matron called me and told the sorry story of how a senior gynaecologist had gone to the Admissions and how shocked he had been. For there were the patients jammed like sardines in a tin. He had ordered their immediate removal back on to beds. "I don't care if they lay two to a bed" he had fumed.

The matron said the doctor had been very angry. He'd looked her in the eye and said, "Matron, if that sister had reported this matter, even to the Daily Dispatch, then we would have had a tremendous scandal on our hands."

You know, I cannot leave off without relating another blazing row, which occurred on night duty. When I came to Frere from Livingstone, their policy was to put new staff on night duty because it was thought that that was the best way to orientate people.

Each morning I had to deliver the night report to the matron, who at the time, was old Miss McGoy.

One day calamity struck when the element of an electric kettle had somehow burned out. It was my lot to report this. From that day on, Miss McGoy repeatedly remarked that Africans are unable to understand the rudiments of electricity. One day she went a little further and added, "There can be good sisters and bad sisters…!"

This remark was to me the red rag to the bull. Then I loosened my tongue to say: "Just like matrons. There can be good matrons and bad. And Miss McGoy... I am tired of hearing about this kettle and about Africans who do not understand electricity. And I'm fed up of hearing about African nurses who like to get pregnant. White nurses get pregnant too and while we have only one little matchbox house in Mdantsane, the white nurses have a flat in town, a house elsewhere and maybe even hide their pregnancies. We can't hide ours in little four-roomed houses." I was so mad that day. She really was a very nasty person.

I remember one day when we were doing rounds with a doctor who was explaining the episiotomy procedure (cutting the lip of the vulva to allow the baby's head an easier way through). We were a mixed group of black and white nurses – this was at Frere Hospital. When he explained how the lip was cut some white nurses pulled their faces and even shuddered in horror. Without a blush the doctor turned and said to them, "Oh, don't worry, that will never be done to ***you***

EDITOR'S NOTE

While visiting a lying-in ward at the Frere Hospital during the course of duty – around 1994 before my secondment to the new Administration at Bisho – I was disturbed to find almost every patient had undergone an episiotomy. I began to enquire of the ward sisters as to why this had been done on such a large scale? Eventually I spotted an obstetrician and approached her with the same question. Her reply shocked me. Speaking in a whisper she said "just a little stitching practice for the intern's sister." If this procedure is placed in a HR perspective it could fall within the HR language and be viewed as "mutilation of the female genitalia." In a political context it could be asked if this is mutilation of black female genitalia.

LAHLEKILE

TRENDS OF THE PIONEERING PERIOD

SOCIAL-POLITICAL BACKDROP

- Females not given adequate education beyond primary school as a rule.
- Social role of girls underpinned by African belief system – marriage, motherhood, submission to male authority.
- Poverty rife in black communities.
- Overt witchcraft and superstition prevailed.
- Traditional healer's most important figures in Africa society.
- Socio-political resistance to the training of black professional nurses.

NURSING EDUCATION

- First trainers Dr Neil Mac Vicar, Eastern Cape, Dr James Mc Cord, Natal - assisted by missionary nurses.
- First training base Victoria Hospital, Alice.
- South African white nurses actively opposed the entry of black nurses into the profession.
- Ethnicity was used to divide nurses.
- Black student nurses were poorly fed.
- Training was basically housekeeping; much emphasis laid on caring by means of touch.
- Little technology in the first 30 years, other than the thermometer.
- Biblical ethics such as submissiveness and humility emphasised.

NURSING PRACTICE

- Salary discrimination and poor salaries an early feature of practice.
- Low status for black nurses within the hierarchical profession.
- Possible origin from two sources, firstly the prevalent belief in black Inferiority; secondly the fact that the training of ward maids preceded that of professional and auxiliary nurses. According to Searle (10:131) the renowned ward maid Anna was "a nurse".
- Non-institutional general nursing ensured a comprehensive service to communities.
- Black nurses were debarred from institutional posts in the first 30 years.
- (Refer map of deployment of Mac Vicar's nurses).
- District nurses were either supervised by health inspectors in magisterial districts or by white matrons who controlled rural area services from hospital offices.
- The 24-hour service was brought in as a mode of practice in rural areas.
- Lack of appropriate transport increased the hardship in practice.
- Nurses of the pioneering period (1906-1930) worked diligently through layers of ignorance, superstition and fears.
- From the 1940's onwards when hospitals posts became available, black nurses came up against doctors who were mostly white males. A master-servant relationship evolved.

THE NURSING STRUGGLE

1913 South African Nurse's Trained Association (SATNA) was formed with a separate branch for blacks entitled ***THE BLACK NURSES'S ASSOCIATION***.

1925 South Africa's first Medical Council was formed with nursing represented by two delegates.

1940's Few black nurses were trained. The reasons were poor schooling and widespread discrimination against black enrolment for the state courses.

CHAPTER 2 - THE MID-CENTURY TRAINEES

PART I - EARLY CHILDHOOD EXPERIENCES

CONTRIBUTORS TO THIS SECTION:

1. Gladys
2. Calabash
3. Noziziwe
4. Mekiwe
5. Pulane
6. Nyameka
7. Asnath
8. Ghalima
9. Mary
10. Nanziwe
11. Constance
12. Nompucuko
13. Maude
14. Linda

GLADYS

My Christian names have no significance being traditional family names but the British surname is another kettle of fish. It came from a grandfather we never knew. He had hailed from England and we've since learned that in London the telephone directory carries an endless list of Arkels.

Well, if you know the history of our country, the British Settlers came out here along with other nationalities – the Cape Mountain Riflemen, the missionaries and so on. Some were good, some bad, others indifferent. Our peer group often talked and joked about it, why many of us had Caucasian features. Some of those men were known to have been offspring of British nobility. They might have been rogues who failed to do well and were then paid by their parents to go overseas.

I once read the story of George Rex of Knysna, a very interesting story that was, though some people tried to deny it. At one time (many years ago) two girls entered our training programme at the Somerset-Hospital in Cape Town. They came from Oudshoorn and bore the surname Rex. The most intriguing thing about their appearance was their long acquiline noses, blue eyes and remarkable resemblance to George Rex of Knysna.

CALABASH

My name is Nomvaba. It is a Xhosa name meaning "Kalabash". A Kalabash is a sour-milk container made of ox-hide, which is cut shaped and sewn into a bag. This bag never empties of milk.

I was born to a family of peasants who were dependent on the fall of rain and the ploughing of land. We lived in the rough, on what could be gleaned from our subsistence economy, so my childhood was harsh.

My father chose this name for me because before my birth there came three sons, which meant that he would have to pay labola three times over. That meant a lot of cows and the real threat that the kalabash would run empty. This threat was so real to those who earned a living from scratching the soil that I suspect it quite unsettled my father's psyche. The birth of a girl brought joy for when she got married his kalabash would again be filled with milk.

NOZIZIWE

My Xhosa name means "Mother of the Nation." I have a proud family history from which I emerge as a fourth generation 'Tsengiwe.' The family had migrated from Keiskamahoek to King Williamstown, Cala and to Umtata. From there we moved to Kimberley and finally Mafeking.

The first generation grandfather was an interpreter at the King Williams Town Magistrate's Court. This ancestor had married a teacher and by the time they settled at Cala our family became known as the first literate arrivals in that dark little corner.

Not only did this couple bring literacy to the locals, they were able to demonstrate healthy agricultural practices too. There were eventually seven sons to provide the skilled manpower for teaching and farming. Meanwhile their father continued his job as court interpreter. I was the daughter of the eldest son after whom an educational institution "The Arthur Training Institute" came to be named. This building was burned down in political riots of the 1980's.

A peculiar tendency was for our family to assimilate Western mores. This is perhaps due to an odd ingredient in the family history. Somewhere along an earlier line a matron of European origin had married in. It was very likely this event that resulted in our capitulation to white culture during colonial rule. It manifested itself in English names being given to all the sons.

LAHLEKILE

Another "claim to fame" for our family was an honour bestowed upon my grandfather a long time ago. It happened when the cartographers came along. They named the vast location that we lived in after him, also a bridge that took us to Indwe where we transported the corn from our farm to be made into flour.

MEKIWE

My name is derived from the concept "circumstances." My paternal grandfather was against my father marrying a girl from the Xhosa clan because he was a Fingo and this was not a tradition in their family.

I was born in Korsten but when I was a year old I was taken over by my maternal grandmother in Uitenhage where I spent the first twelve years of my life. Being an "only child" in their home, I had everything that I could want since both my parents were working.

I attended school at a Methodist missionary establishment not very far from home. We walked the short distance in groups wearing tackies (sneakers) because shoes were reserved for church only.

Those years we were educated under the Good Hope system, which was fathoms better than the awful "Bantu Education" brought in under the architect of apartheid, (the late) Dr Hendrik Verwoerd.

One happy memory of school years was the generosity of the farmers of Kirkwood and the surrounding areas. They donated pockets of succulent oranges to the school and everybody - including our teachers - benefited from this goodwill.

CALABASH

I grew up in a village called Jwaxa Location in Middledrift. Despite my poverty-stricken background I was a high achiever at school. Up to secondary level I went through three different schools. We had to walk backwards and forwards and did not know of shoes.

The first school was in the village but at a point far from home. The second was double the distance. To get there we had to leave without breakfast long before the sun began to sting. En route we traversed a tangle of road and undulating hills and had dust blown up in our faces from passing cars. If we were late we were given corporal punishment.

NOZIZIWE

My schooling proper began at Mafeking at the Roman Catholic Mission. I became a member of the "Sunbeam" group. An outstanding event was for me to be chosen as the "Sunbeam" who had to present a bouquet of flowers to the English Queen (now grandmother to Prince Charles) during the Royal Family's visit to our country.

PULANE

I grew up in a large religious family from my mother's side. My father grew up in a very harsh environment in a place called Ramupedi near Kuruman on the outskirts of the North West.

LAHLEKILE

He often related stories of the chieftainship and the power positions and the witchcraft that governed their lives. My father so disliked this lifestyle that in his youth he ran away to Postmasburg out of fear that eventually his entire family might be annihilated by the witchcraft.

My mother's family was much admired. They were raised in a civilised manner, more modern than traditional. Their father hailed from Groenwater. My maternal family were deprived of their land, forcibly removed from Groenwater to a horribly sandy place called Rietfontein, far out in the Northern Cape.

Relatives told of how, when they first set foot there, how unbearably dreary the place had been, how degradingly filthy with snakes crawling all over. They nicknamed the place "Sandfontein". Thus were Blacks permanently domiciled outside the towns of South Africa. Nowadays people are able to make land claims where they feel they've been deprived of their land by the former regime but this came too late for my folks.

GHALIMA

I was named after my grandmother. In Islam we believe in breast-feeding but my mother had poor lactation so my Granny was my "wet nurse."

I was born in District Six, schooled at Ashley Street Primary and then went on to Trafalgar High. The most shocking event of my childhood was our forced removal from District Six. The issue raised media attention, lots of hype around the world, but we who lived there suffered the most appalling stress. I was still a growing girl but thinking about it even now, well it strikes a vibrant nerve.

The mass removal made everything rush at us all at once. I can remember running around like a mouse on a treadmill. District Six had a well-integrated business community, its commerce a ceaseless tremor of activity. Jewish and Indian people had shops side by side. When this aspect of our lives fell under the political axe, the pain was sharp in the collective heart, as if we'd been stung by wasps.

A feature of District Six – on the negative side – was the skolly element. Those gangsters had worked the ploy of intimidation to a fine art. They struck fear into the hearts of everyone and could intimidate the law enforcers too. They could stick a knife into someone without a twitch of conscience, but they demonstrated a measure of respect for local residents.

Admittedly District Six had numerous slum areas and alleys but those could have been upgraded. The Boer government had no business breaking up a cohesive, multi-cultural and entirely colour-blind community such as ours.

One of the amazing acts of neighbourliness in our community life was the religious tolerance. My family lived in Albert Street with the mosque across the road from us. Two doors away lived the Benjamin family who were Christians.

When it came to Ramadan they knew it was a time of fasting for us. No one would appear near us eating as much as a crust of bread, so much did they respect our religion. With the evening call to prayer, the Christian children would melt off the streets while we were in the mosque or in our homes at prayer.

This is how we grew up and this is the wonderful social system that had to be ripped apart by the one-dimensional vision of the Boer-government.

NOZIZIWE

Our final voluntary migration took us to Mafeking where one by one, segments of the family followed. Eventually a massive resettlement occurred. My sister remarked that we were so like the "Indian" people. When one comes, the others simply follow.

All our adult males became landowners even if it meant two jobs, teaching and farming. My grandfather had pushed them in that direction. So we witnessed the spread of our settlement, like an octopus lying under the sun-yellow horizon. The place came to be known as "Union Park" and to this day our official family home remains there. However our idyllic existence was rudely disturbed.

With sickened hearts we were forced to sell our land when the boere (Nationalist Government) came to power. In two shakes of a duck's tail they came up with convincing arguments (to themselves) as to why Africans could not farm there. Two decades later gold was discovered. A relative wrote to keep us informed. She told of massive pieces of machinery being off-loaded on to our farmland.

In the interim my father had decided to retrace his footsteps to Cala in the Eastern Cape. His father had very fortunately made a will securing his erven in Cala. This land had been hired out for years by a great-aunt of ours and today that land bears ownership for my grandfather's descendants.

NYAMEKA

I was born in the "Red location" in Port Elizabeth. It was the only location in New Brighton at the time. I grew up with my maternal grandparents, an institutionalised cultural practice of the time. My mother had many siblings so I grew up under the compelling warmth of an extended family.

We were Christians. Everything was imbued with faith and spirit. My grandparents were milkers. In those days things were very cheap, no malignant VAT. You could buy half a loaf of bread for a tickey (3-pence) a big piece of meat for one-and-sixpence, probably the equivalent of our ten-cent piece today.

In the Red Location it was the custom to brew "kaffir beer" as a commercial enterprise. This was well organised. The area was divided up into blocks with each block getting a turn on a weekly basis. As young children we were engaged in a flurry of activity, purchasing mealie meal and other ingredients for the "aunties". Our legs pranced high and fast in this cause.

There were frantic arguments amongst ourselves as we stood in the warmth of the African sun. "This block is mine". "No, no, that aunty belongs to me." All to ensure a legitimate entry into the crammed shop a little distance away. The lucky ones would savour its treasures and receive "basalla" (free sweets) when their purchases were made. It was a street event, which added a fillip to our lives.

Throughout childhood years we were taught entrancing norms and values. This created an interlocking social milieu for us. Older adults were reverently addressed as "Mama" or "Tata". We would stand up when visitors entered the house and automatically depart for the kitchen to boil water either on a primus stove or on the massive Dover if the fire was going.

These coal-and-wood stoves were left to the children to clean over weekends. We had to take out all those iron plates with a poker to wash off the soot. This was dirty, arduous work but the children in the community accepted it as natural that it should be their task.

Before bringing in the tea you prepared for the visitors you would ask, "May I come in please Mama?" Mother would sit up, feign delight and say, "Oh, have you brought some tea for Aunty who is visiting Mama? Well, come in child."
We owe our generation of parents a debt of gratitude for the culture they passed on to us in this way.

ASNATH

This name – in my father's view – came from the Bible. She was the mother of Joseph, I think. I grew up in the Northern Transvaal in the Soutpansberg area. This had become the political constituency of (the late) Dr Andries Treurnicht the leader of the Conservative Party in Afrikaner politics.

I lived in a village – a mission community under the auspices of Swiss missionaries. All the members of the Epharate Church lived in this village surrounded by mountains and enfolded by magnificent acacia trees.

The scenery was breathtaking especially in spring and summer. The grey mountain peaks looked magical in the afternoon sun and would change from grey-mauve to purple with the fall of twilight. On a clear night everything looked serene under a phosphorescent moon.

With the advent of spring the grass would sprout bright green. You could sniff the spring from the rich earth. Truly we were cocooned in a rhythm of life as steady and predictable as the seasons.

My mother came from a village in the Pietersburg area where there were no schools for Africans in that part of the world so she remained illiterate. Nevertheless she was a woman of above-average intelligence.

In those days, families chose spouses for their children. My father was a priest and his parents sent him in her direction. Fortunately Cupid's bow struck home.

My mother occupied herself by running a little dairy, which she owned. She was never too busy to beam at us, her expression flooded with affection. She had a good head for business because she also sold large clay pots, her eyes dark with palpitating excitement whenever she traded a clay pot for the clink of hard currency.

We were six children in the brood with me being the only girl. Really, I take my hat off to my mother who succeeded in educating every one of us through sheer hard work. I further admire her for her exquisite cooking skills, which she passed on to us. One of my brothers became a chef, another an agricultural officer, all of us became something and I think she deserves a crown of some sort for that. I shall never forget her endearing smile and the rustle of her cotton dress as she moved with pure African grace and dignity.

PART 2 - THE PRACTICE YEARS

PRELUDE

Regina kicked off her duty shoes and sipped gratefully on the delicious cup of Rooibos tea handed to her by Aunt Emily. "Gosh, this is a moment to be cherished" she said, smacking her lips.

Aunt Emily – spry, brown and fidgety – sat in a rattan chair to resume the crochet work she had put aside to make the tea. "You girls work too hard and for far too little money," she grumbled good-naturedly.

They sat in amicable silence each wrapped in their own thoughts. Regina began to feel the ache ease from her feet and mused, "Whenever will I enjoy such leisure as her? She makes retirement seem like a dream." As she felt her self drift into a delicious, lethargic doze the thought emerged that soon this bliss would be disturbed by a knock on the door. She had no idea how true that would be, nor how soon a benevolent fate was to plunge her into an obstetric nightmare.

All too soon there was a hammering on the door, which fell as an assault on her ears. She rushed to open first the fly mesh then the heavy teak door and found a complete stranger, a rag-bag kind of person standing on the raffia mat with an air of urgency. "Come quickly Nurse, there is a woman in great trouble up in the kloof."

"Who is she?" asked Regina with an air of resignation. "I don't know. She is kneeling down and has covered herself with a blanket; there is a young woman with her."

Regina flew in his footsteps. Her leg muscles were strong from the great distances she had to walk each day. Getting to the kloof was hard though, walking uphill against the undulating landscape. She felt the cold morning air bite into her cheeks.

Soon her eyes spotted the woman and her heart contracted in fright. "Oh no, not No Eleven?" she thought. What bad luck was stalking her all of a sudden? No Eleven was a grande multip (a woman who has had many babies) now presenting with a multiple pregnancy. Her case was complicated and she had to see the doctor every two weeks. She was due to be X-rayed at the very next visit. Regina felt her brain ticking over. It was as though a time bomb had been placed in her hands and she was not quite sure what to do with it.

"What is she doing in the kloof?" she asked the man who was striding ahead of her with the manner of a mountaineer. He wore cheap, baggy, shapeless clothes. She felt an invigorating tension build up in her mind. He spoke crisply, "She had gone to the kloof to relieve herself."

The edge of panic nudged at Regina. For a moment she stood still and bowed her face into cupped hands. She was thinking, "She must have ruptured her membranes and if that is so then she has plunged me into the quicksand's of midwifery. What am I to do?"

At last they reached No Eleven who held out a coffee-coloured arm the moment she saw Regina. "Take me home Nurse, please Nurse, I want to go home" she blubbered hoarsely. There were tears oozing from her popping eyes and running down the puffed cheeks. Regina made a hasty calculation casting her eyes around the immediate locale. She decided that "home" was definitely nearer than the clinic and beckoned the man closer for assistance.

Together they propped the patient – whose legs threatened to give under her – up into a standing position. She instructed the young woman standing by dumb with fright, to hasten to fetch her midwifery bag at her house and they then began the tortuous journey from the kloof to the patient's house about half a kilometre away, perched on another hill.

The walk was timeless. It was the kind of day that made you want to go running and leaping towards the horizon. Instead, they were reigned in by the arduous pace of a woman in the final stages of multiple birth. Regina's heart was hammering so hard she thought it would explode.

When at last they reached the door of the house No Eleven managed just a few tottering steps inside when she sank on the floor like a sack of potatoes suddenly falling loose. Immediately she positioned herself in the lithotomy position and promptly began pushing very hard while her lips split and her teeth grated on something.

Regina summoned a reserve of energy and galvanised herself into action. Rolling up her sleeves she shouted for hot water, jumped to support a protruding head, then catching the meconium-stained infant just in time before the force of birth could jet-propel the little body on to the ground.

The infant was lifeless and she had barely cut and clamped the cord when she had to race to attend to the second delivery. She felt a chill rise to the top of her stomach when barely 15 minutes after the second infant a third was ready to come. Silence drifted in the thickened room when the realisation hit home that none of the babies were alive. When Regina indicated that a fourth birth was imminent there was a murmur of shock and approbation.

Regina's brow was laced with drops of perspiration. Her mind rioted as she delivered the last little mite. This was unbelievable. How could four babies come out of the birth canal with such rapid rhythm virtually without pause, tragically without life? The routine task of cutting and clamping the umbilical cord suddenly turned into a nightmarish job; her hands were shaking, her fingers suddenly turned to rubber.

All the while the mother was groaning in anguish. Regina could understand upon sober reflection that this was wholly feasible. There were the twin complications of malnutrition and maternal age. Add to that the lack of qualitative obstetric care. Then spontaneous abortion became all too possible. Bit it was still moving to witness the glittery tears springing from the mother's eyes.

The neighbours were busy as bees alongside Regina. They were preparing a mat for her lying-in period, clucking sympathetically as they worked. Regina made the patient comfortable on the mat; they drank the hot tea brought in from next-door. Everyone by that time needed the relief of a hot beverage.

Meanwhile the male relatives were preparing a small mass grave outside, some distance from the house. The tiny little bodies were put to rest in a sombre atmosphere under a pile of wooden crosses. The father was shaking his head mutely. He had not been dealt a good hand of cards, Regina mused, as she stood outside sipping tea while watching the proceedings.

As far as her practice was concerned this had been a momentous experience. It had had the ingredients of drama and she knew that her performance had been a credible one.

REGINA SPEAKS

A personal crisis hit us as a group of final year trainees at Frere Hospital. We were greatly offended and diminished by the racial discrimination especially when we had to subject ourselves to junior white nurses whenever our seniors were off-duty. In fact we felt embarrassed and humiliated by this blatant racist practice.

One day we finalists decided to bring our complaint to the Hospital Board. An appointment was made and our agenda accepted. Our elected spokesperson presented our cause for complaint after which there was a pause, a long moment stretched thin and taut. Then the superintendent, a man whom we greatly respected, rose. We held our breath collectively when he cleared his throat and began to address us in a low voice with neither approval nor exhortation.

He said, "You have a valid cause for complaint ladies, but the hospital also has a genuine reason for acting as it does. We come from different cultures, environments and traditions. Some of you still ignore and pass by a dripping tap instead of tightening it because you in the rural areas do not pay for water but fetch it from a river.

When some of you go to a kit-room at night you switch on the light but one or the other forgets to put it off because you do not appreciate the cost involved. A white child is taught from early childhood about these things costing money, even if it is government money. After all, governments get money from taxpayers and that is you and me. The fact is that even an unborn white child is equipped with a higher degree of intelligence than children of other races…."

We felt sick. In fact I was appalled to hear our people so disdainfully described, to witness the bigotry of a man we had so respected. Despair and helplessness locked our lips. There was nothing that we could do except put pride in our back pockets and continue working under the humiliation of white "superiority" something no power on earth could make us believe.

ASNATH

As far as I am concerned we were plunged into crisis from the day we commenced training. This was in 1941 at the Elm Hospital in Northern Transvaal. It was as though we were convicts condemned to hard labour –

cleaning, scrubbing, shining, sluicing, as well as basic nursing and bedside care.

Numerous difficulties arose to sour our lives. As student nurses the socio-economic aspects were most appalling. Can you imagine the paltry income of 5 shillings a month? That was daylight robbery, which made our lives one of continuous passive unhappiness.

The uniforms were atrocious. We looked worse than disconsolate waifs. Old uniforms were collected in Switzerland and we had no choice but to wear them whether they had been patched or not. Often we looked and felt like medieval nuns.

As far as accommodation was concerned, my heart shrivelled in my breast when first I saw our living quarters. We were housed, in as far as a roof covered our heads, but for the rest everything was very, very threadbare. In my wildest imagination I could not have conjured up a more abysmal scenario.

The meals were especially abominable. I cannot find words to describe what we were given to eat except that it demonstrated an utter lack of care on the part of Europeans for the welfare of African people. The inadequate diet goaded us almost beyond endurance; our every nerve shrieked for relief. You could say that if the physical accommodation was the wound then the food issue was an explosion of pus. Furthermore the educative aim of the place had been completely overlooked.

Another acute social problem, which reared its head, was that we were treated according to some military mode. If you were found walking with a boy your lungs clutched for oxygen because soon you would be hauled on the carpet for strict rebuke and punishment. It gave one a sense of being pushed aside by totally unfair rhetoric. You would stand there like a child while shaken up by a paroxysm of emotion far removed from childish feelings. In fact it felt as though you were in a bad dream toppling through space to a dim, silent, bottomless pit and all the time you were aching to come to wakefulness. So as young people we were deprived of the basic right of freedom of association.

MEKIWE

My first crisis occurred during training. It was an experience that carried an element of fun out of the solemnity and finality of death. As junior nurses we were expected to lie out corpses and transport these to the mortuary. This was a task which the porters (white at that time) would never assist nurses with. They were barely able to raise more than an antagonistic interest.

On a particular day we had to tackle the difficult duty of laying out a lady patient who had passed away during the early hours. We came on duty fresh as daisies and it was grim to be confronted with a corpse as large as St Mary's Cathedral. Four of us were assigned to the procedure due to the unusual size of the body.

With due respect we carried out the grim duty then two of us galloped to the porter's office where we found these white employees sitting down smoking. We knew that they would not lift a finger to help us, playing little more than a backroom role at the mortuary.

When we reached the ward with the "death trolley" in tow, we faced the horrendous task of having to lift and lay the body on the stretcher.

Now I'm not sure whether the trolley was on a level with the bed; all I know is that we had to lift her up before placing her down.

Our original four attempted to do the impossible. After all we were young and full of animal vitality. The fact that we were unable to perform this feat caused a ruckus in the ward. We then leaped around with tremendous energy searching for help in other wards.

Our attitude of urgency persuaded ward sisters to pull in their horns. They remonstrated that we were to leave behind at least one junior nurse to hold the fort for them. By this means we eventually harvested almost our entire block for the single task confronting us. It was like getting a team of frail beach models to lift a dead whale out of the sea at low tide.

After a truly monumental performance we were able to get the body on to the trolley. It was decided that eight nurses in all could proceed to the mortuary. This was a sight for sore eyes, since normally it is done by two. The public very likely gained the impression that we were transporting a VIP of sorts.

At the mortuary a fresh crisis stared us in the face in that the trays were chock-full. Putting our heads together we planned our way around the situation. All the while I had the feeling that I must not become affected, being face-to-face with death.

LAHLEKILE

I said, "Look, let's take the lower shelf because that man there is lighter because he was younger." We managed to put his corpse on the floor blowing much hot air while doing so. Then began a titanic tug-of-war with the one that we had brought that would have put an Olympic team to shame.

We began to lift, tug, push and pull with all our might, huffing and puffing. Being less in number we were clearly hobbled by the ton-weight. With caps askew, bruising hands, straining backs, we nevertheless managed to deposit our corpse on the bottom shelf, laughing all the way at our own puny strength.

The moment this was done we collapsed in a heap, convulsed with laughter, feeling the collective strength fizzling out. But we soon realised with horror that we were sharing space with another being who had slipped off the coil of life. His enshrouded body was a grim reminder that our ordeal was far from over.

Inspecting the shelves on tiptoe we discovered that one upper shelf had three small children's' bodies on it. No doubt everybody's heart leaped in commiseration for this tragedy as mine did. It was such a crude reminder of how precious life really is.

We removed the little bodies to the floor and in more sombre frame of mind commenced the replacement of the young man's body, not without great exertion once again.

No matter how we tried we were unable to find space for the children's bodies. In the end, our nerves sapped with physical exhaustion, we did the only thing possible to us.

Without a backward glance we took ourselves off in long-legged strides leaving behind a bizarre situation for the porters to solve. One nurse had placed the little bodies in a neat row; another had ensured that the nametags attached to their big toes were right side up. More we could not do.

NYAMEKA

Around 1987 a crisis occurred in casualty where I was working. A Sister Swartz was in charge. There was a patient, Connie Varies (name changed), who had a goitre and was being attended to by Dr Maasdorp who at this time was doing ENT. Dr Maasdorp had ordered Logo's iodine 10 minums TDS. A student-nurse took the Logo's iodine and a minum measure along to Sister Swarts to have it checked. This was one of casualty's busiest moments.

Full of gush and bubble she then proceeded – without ascertaining how this was to be administered – to drop 10 minums with a pipette into Connie's eyes. The patient recoiled as though her eyes had been scalded. Since the treatment was prescribed "TDS" the diligent student repeated it at noon.

When I came on duty at 2pm I discovered the patient in the ablution quarters. She was trembling, standing with her head down and seemed to be suffocated by pain, grief and rage. "What's wrong Connie?" I asked, truly appalled.

"Sister, the nurse keeps putting stuff into my eyes and it's burning like fire and now I cannot even open my eyes." Her features were pitched into a deep contortion.

I scrutinised the doctor's orders, went along to Sr. Swartz and said softly, "Sister will you check with me please? Look what the doctor has written, yet the student-nurse claims that you approved that she should put this iodine into the patient's eyes?"

Sister Swartz's face instantly darkened from ruddy to plum-coloured. Holding her head like someone demented she hopped up and down in agitation screaming hoarsely, "Here, Here, sy lieg! Ek het nie so ges nie, sy lieg!" (Lord, Lord, she's lying! I did not say that, she's lying!") When she called the student to our presence the sound of her voice lashed like a whip. She was ready to tear the student into shreds.

The patient meanwhile had to endure the loss of sight, and having her eyes painfully glued shut. It was an era when South African patients were not aware of their legal powers.

Dr Maasdorp consulted all the eye-specialists that he could think of, to reverse what had been done to the patient. They rallied round, sustaining him emotionally. He sacrificed lunch and supper that day to sit in immobility and silence beside the patient. It seemed that a leaden melancholy had laid him low.

Fortunately things improved to the point that the damage was reversed and the patient fully recovered. Doctor Maasdorp took the matter up with his colleagues who were advising him what not to do. So nothing happened which could have caused an official tremor in Dr Swartz's domain. Our relief was palpable. When Connie responded to her surroundings as if nothing untoward had happened, the grin on Dr Maasdorp's face was a kilometre wide.

MEKIWE

An unforgettable crisis occurred during my second year of training when I was assigned to the eye theatre. The patient was a young man who had been stabbed in the right eye, which was now to be enucleated (taken out).

Normally all theatre staff were conversant with the surgical procedure and all the checks that go along with it. Most unfortunately on this day the black sister who was supposed to scrub up was nowhere to be seen. In fact she arrived on duty later than was expected.

What complicated the situation more was the common knowledge that the surgeon who was to perform the operation and the white sister then deputising, were having a sizzling affair. She had breezed in, animal vitality communicating itself and I watched her drape herself nonchalantly in theatre garb, doing the same for the surgeon while basking in his attention. There was a kind of electric anticipation between them.

During the checking procedure it was discovered that one bottle was depleted of fluid, which would be needed. The sister who had already scrubbed up ran to the dispensary basket that was kept outside the theatre door. She grabbed a replacement bottle, returned to the theatre, but failed to check the bottle with anyone. At that point a warning pulse began to throb in me.

The surgeon drew up from this bottle and injected the fluid into the patient's eye. The patient recoiled in pain.

Two things happened then. I ran to the window-will to check the bottle she had placed there. I could not recognise the contents as the same as that in the previous bottle though I could read clearly what was labelled on it. I found myself in an instant conflict of emotions.

At the same time the surgeon asked the patient, "What is happening Thomas?" He uttered a desperate screech, something like: "It's so painful doctor, I can die!" The surgeon somehow regarded this as a joke for he said to the sister, "No, tell him it's a good job, good job." This set them off laughing; for them life was an absolute breeze. That hurt deep into my innermost being.

The surgeon then proceeded to inject a further requirement of the same fluid into the eye. This time the patient's face distorted into an indescribable grimace of pain. Within seconds he collapsed with cardiac arrest. He had been more gravely affected than anyone could possibly have realised.

At that moment the sister who was supposed to have taken the table, entered the theatre. In the confusion of the hubbub she had no idea what was happening. In seconds flat the patient died. Everyone was stunned and inarticulate.

We were called to the office of Miss Uys the Chief matron. First she shouted at the black sister, "Why were you not at your post taking over the table as you were supposed to have done?" Then she turned to me in all her sternness: "Why didn't you see that it was the wrong fluid?"

With my heart beating in my throat I said, "No Matron, not until the patient screamed the first time because that sister didn't check the bottle with me." She barked "And what did you do?" I said, "I tried to draw their attention Matron because when I saw what was written on the label I knew it was the wrong fluid, but they were laughing and could not see or hear what I wanted to tell them."

Miss Uys then poured a torrent of denunciations and snide observations in my face. Somehow I realised that her attitude stemmed from an inescapable dilemma. She immediately punished the two of us by having all our off-duty time taken away. Furthermore we were confined to the Nurses' Home outside duty until further notice. Naturally I smarted under the injustice.

Meanwhile the matter was passed to higher levels of the national provincial administration. Inevitably the day came when the big guns arrived on our doorstep to institute an Enquiry. As a witness I moved up the stairs in a daze when called.

With dreadful heavy heart I became aware of the matron awaiting me half-way up the stairs and I want to show you what she did to me: (demonstrates the laying on of hands for the purpose of shaking up physically the other person).

MEKIWE CONTINUES

All the while she was shaking me in a paroxysm of rage she spoke in staccato tones: "You-must-not-tell-lies…what-happened-in-theatre-was-not-as-you-told-it-the-other-day." I became aware of sweat running down her face.

Upon entering the room I was trembling with trepidation remembering how the black sister had cried bucketsful under the threats of the chief matron. Yet when I stepped over the threshold I began to have a feeling of ease. There were no others besides the men from head-office and they were gentlemen, one could see at a glance.

In the trusting atmosphere that they created, I was able to outline the facts. They wanted to know precisely what I had seen on the bottle the sister had substituted. I spelled out the truth, that it had been ADENALIN I:1000 IN TARTRATE. Being doctors themselves these doctors dropped their heads in shock. One said, "Oh my God." There was no need for me to add the hurtful scene about the laughter. Already the crime of neglect had been illuminated as though in neon lights.

There were no streams of questions. All they said, was, "Thank you very much Nurse for having been alert." It was the low ebb of a weary fairy-tale.

In the aftermath during which the surgeon and the sister were suspended, Matron Uys descended on me with all her screeching might. "Ja, you were the one who opened the can of worms at the Enquiry. You saw in the dark theatre what had happened." Whenever she had cause to speak to me her face was set, lips twitching, eyes darting left and right. My truthfulness had set up a festering in her.

GLADYS

'I never had any difficulties during my working years, not with posts or anything else. I watched others vie for positions and saw colleagues grapple with professional jealousies but I never had such difficulties. However my involvement with SANA was something else.

Those years we had to fight, fight, fight for equal rights and equal opportunities. Conference after conference we used to argue and fight – oh dear, send in resolutions and stand there for hours, pleading our cause and the answer was always: *THIS IS THE WHITE SALARY. THIS IS THE COLOURED AND INDIAN SALARY. THIS IS THE BLACK SALARY. The discrepancy* in the salary structure was what used to eat us. Man it really ate into our souls.

Came 1957 when *SANA* was forced to sign what the Government expected of them. In other words they had to bring apartheid into the Nursing Act and specify the "white" group, the "coloured and Indian" group, the "black" group. This was really too much for us. And in a sense it killed something deep down in a person, in those of us who were sensitive about our repression. And who wasn't? Look what came out of all this.

Year after year after year this went on. That was besides pressure from head office pleading with us to attend SANA meetings. Before this Act was changed we used to attend meetings in common with the whites and blacks in Cape Town. I still remember the Metropolitan Church Hall where the meetings were mainly held. Once a month we used to meet there.

LAHLEKILE

Came this *thing* and it just killed off every professional spark, everything. It was very sad. I had a great liking for Doreen Radloff (Do you know that she is gravely ill at the moment with something affecting her mental faculties?) I remember telling them in no uncertain terms how we felt about the apartheid in nursing. Afterwards Doreen and I walked together to the car and talked more about it. She explained that their hands were tied behind their backs. "They hated the apartheid too but they had no way of circumventing the law."

I suppose the professional crisis I faced was the outcome of all this really. In 1957 I was on my way to a *SANA* meeting. I was walking across St George's Street when a restraining hand passed across my vision and a voice said with a note of urgency,

"Don't go Miss Arkle, don't go!" that was when the nurses decided for the first time to boycott the *SANA* meetings. I said to my adversary, "Man, I only want to go and listen." Those were crisis times when we were deeply hurt by all that was happening.

Then in 1969 I was confronted by a huge mob consisting of trained nurses, students, and health workers. I had no idea what their intention was, whether to hurt me physically or not but I didn't feel that *I* was responsible for their paltry salaries. I became aware only of a torrent of mob anger coming at me in waves. No, I didn't feel overwhelmed or scared, just so angry that the mob should have approached *me*, surely a pathologically inaccurate target for their anger?

At the grassroots level we nurses were powerless. The administration claimed to be powerless too. They had to knuckle down – this I believe – to the Government for whom apartheid was a diamond-hard state objective. Yet this was something that the broad mass of nurses palpably disbelieved.

Many of the girls called us "Government stooges" because they had decided to turn their backs on *SANA*, to drop everything, to resist. But we had decided to continue the struggle from within, to fight. Their accusation that we were government stooges was one, which I found indigestible. They do not know of the anguish, the pain, the suffering that we endured for the sake of keeping our profession alive.

We were the nurses who picked up the reigns and chartered a course through legal and ethical minefields. We steered the profession through all the political upheavals which impinged from outside. I feel that we are all entitled to our disparate opinions and you cannot force people to think the way you want them to. I get impatient and angry even though I sound eminently reasonable.

EDITOR'S NOTE:

What was clear to Gladys and her peers even in 1957 was that the system had placed nursing on a runaway engine. Today we see apartheid sink below the waters and no doubt we shall watch it disappear without trace, at least from the statute book. Still, if contemporary nurses are rising towards the apex of a liberated profession then Gladys and her peers were at the slope of the same pyramid, fighting to clear the way in the context of their time.

LAHLEKILE

MARY

A crisis occurred one day that I shall never forget. I am not going to mention names nor identify the place. It was a situation where members of the public had been shot and it had nothing to do with politics or the police.

This incident resembled a mini war. It happened in 1991 in a very small town. A gang of thieves had held up a woman while she was transporting money to the bank in the presence of an armed escort. Apparently they had left their shop and were en route to the car when a robber walked up to them and demanded that they hand over the money.

At that moment a petrol truck came by driven by a young (white) man who intervened. He was shot and killed on the spot. Meanwhile the lady was trying to shield her armed guard who had been wounded in his arm. When I saw him he stood stock still with mouth open and lips frozen. By the time we got there in our mobile van the noise was such that I expected my eardrums to be blown to pieces.

Scores of people were bleeding, lying moribund. Onlookers were as thick as a swarm of bees. The robbers by then had reeled out of control shooting aimlessly in an exploding flash of flames. Someone was caught in the neck, others in various parts of the body. There was blood everywhere; I nearly gagged in the street. We may have stood with outwardly grave composure but actually we were bewildered, not knowing where to go.

What followed next happened automatically. I jammed myself amongst the black patients and my colleague fled to the white side. We sprang into action and did what we could. There were no words to rub together; everything was reduced to sweaty silence. The white man who had intervened was dead so she ran to those whites that were still alive. I did the same to the blacks. Really, we didn't plan it that way; each ran to those whom we could best communicate with.

Apartheid stalked out every footstep.

I was working at a clinic where there were two entrances. The front entrance was reserved for whites and the back for blacks. Should a black dare go to the front entrance he or she was at risk of being chased away as though a wild animal on the prowl. "Can't you see that this side is for whites only?" Without fail the white nurse would remonstrate with the black client. We black nurses were thoroughly demoralised as were the people of our community.

But one day a new member of staff who happened to be young, politically enlightened and *black* confronted the white sister who had apartheid embedded in her psyche. I must admit that our generation of "old" nurses rarely had the nerve to stick up for our rights. We tended to tolerate the status quo. The little ones coming after us are different and thank God for that.

One day a black was again rudely chased away from the front door and this new sister locked horns with the white nurse, cutting her down to size. She made me feel so lekker man (so nice). With a light gleaming in her eye the new nurse said, "What difference does it make? What makes you so much better than blacks? White as you are, that woman is better than you by far because you are such a rude person, you have no respect for her age or her personal dignity…"

I do not wish to repeat every word of the altercation but I could see that her telling-off had hit home. The white sister was mortally wounded and no longer could she stand on firm ground.

In fact soon after that incident she decided to leave. To be quite honest that sister had not been particularly kind to her own people either. She had somehow earned a reputation for handling patients harshly. Anyway her departure brought a breath of fresh air to the daily grind and things went much better after that.

NANZIWE

A crisis hit me at Livingstone in 1968. It was a time when all the white sisters and matrons used to take the weekends off, leaving the running of the hospital – including the maternity department – to the blacks. One white matron remained on call.

A flood of huge dimensions broke out of the heavens at about 9:45. Half the staff had gone to tea and phoned to say they could not return because the tunnel was flooded out. I suddenly had to put my closest fears into mental recesses.

Then Maternity phoned to say that the bottom floor was flooded out and they did not know where to take the babies, since now the nursery too was affected and in an acute situation of crisis.

To add to the intense horror the lifts started to burst into flame, an acrid smell creeping into our nostrils. In I.C.U. we had patients on oxygen so that by then anxiety was stalking me like an enemy bent on confrontation. Being the supervisor in charge I not only had to don my thinking cap but press the alert button too. When I phoned the white matron on call she responded (with built-in condescension) that she could not come since her car would be flooded under. Incredulous at her reply I felt my hope shatter like ice crystals.

Most immediately I had to figure out whether to stop the oxygen or take the orthopaedic patients down via the fire escape since the lifts were burning. I think there was a patient who delivered in the ambulance outside but that was one of the multiple problems, which the medical and nursing staff handled with impeccable professional calm.

At first I was able to keep the superintendent informed. He said, "Take keys, go to the kitchen and give everybody whatever food there is." After 10am communication was suddenly cut so we lost our contact with him too. I then set the pace for an action-planned operation for the survival of the patients and our selves.

By some miracle there were no diabetics to contend with. A hum, as of a disturbed hive of bees filled the air as we grabbed bread, cheese, eggs, whatever we could lay our hands on, and all the patients ate the same food. I was on duty for 12 hours that day and could never ever forget that flood.

Another crisis occurred in 1952, this time political. This was the time of the Defiance Campaign when blacks were trampled and crushed by the state. There was tension between the doctors and nurses because police were shooting left, right and centre. The conflict arose because we were required to take patients' names, those who had bullets. They would then be arrested and become prisoners.

The nurses were naturally protective of their people and were deeply wounded by the arrests. Meanwhile the doctors were protective of the system. They showed not a spasm of feeling. By the same token I myself was unable to raise a modicum of patriotism within me.

What further repelled me was seeing the police chain our people to their beds. They appeared to be in a political time warp after all, this was hardly the time of Jan Van Riebeeck when people were trapped, chained and whipped without restraint. (Reference 18). The job of the police was to guard the patients, not to chain them like captive animals. It was clear to me that their humanity had fallen into ashes.

A third crisis was when a student nurse – again over a weekend when there were no whites and I was super-anxious that nothing should go wrong – when this nurse committed a crime against a helpless patient.

It happened that in the paediatric ward a patient had messed himself. The nurse was so furious that instead of cleaning the infant she took him to the sluice room, opened the hot and cold taps and pushed him under. I remember that it was a coloured baby. My response was to immediately suspend her from duty.

The Nursing Council of course had a disciplinary hearing and her name was scratched from the Register.

Finally on the matter of crises, just to show how indescribably sad nursing often is, it happened one day that a wrong lung had been accidentally operated upon. The patient was placed in a side ward and we had to monitor the death.

CONSTANCE

Your question about a professional crisis takes me back to 1952 in East London. That was the time of the Defiance Campaign when political upheaval occurred and blacks were shot like flies. I was on duty for almost 24 hours because when news of the riot in Bantu Street broke, I went to Casualty to render assistance.

I shall never forget the volcanic atmosphere at the hospital that fatal Sunday. Every second had the familiarity of a nightmare. People were coming in by ambulance with bullet wounds, some groaning, others moribund. Many were drunk, being free to imbibe on Sundays.

A very shocking thing occurred at the hospital. Before my very eyes the patients were kicked into Casualty. The police threw them out of the vans onto the ground from where they were rolled in and kicked as though they were bundles of dirty laundry. I saw it happen, so no one must come along to deny this. It was a sight that made me shrivel into myself.

It was not only from the police. There were some white doctors and nurses (amongst the many good doctors and nurses) who were manhandling the patients too. I was a witness to that as well. Around us blood was running in a thick, sludgy river. We worked non-stop even while witnessing the great outrage described above, which I saw.

While my hands worked, danger signals were flashing in my mind. It still comes back so clearly. In my heart there was a terrible constriction because of the shocking treatment my people were getting. My eyes were of course smarting with pain and frustration but I continued working as though made of steel. It seemed at the time as though my chest had been bisected.

Around us there was a profusion of movement, from the police, ambulance drivers, security people, health personnel; everything was reduced to chaos. The patients were not treated as human beings by many of the whites and that is one experience that I shall carry with me into eternity.

Another crisis, which affected my whole life was of course my detention without trial.

First and foremost, let me say that I always believe that I am free to do as I like in my home and in the vicinity where I live.

So I got involved in the Civic Association, which is a community organisation. I did what I thought was best for the community to which I belong.

Our priority at the time was to take education out of the crisis situation it was in through the abysmal lack of schools. Space was needed urgently to accommodate the large numbers of Duncan Village children thirsting for education as desert vegetation does for water.

We were interested in low-cost buildings and every effort was made to allow for schools that could be swiftly erected.

I was amongst the people who went to see the sample structures at Breidbach but to my surprise, when we came back, the structures which were put up not far from the new housing area called Gompo town, did not resemble what we saw and approved at Breidback.

I was one member of a delegation who voiced the community's objection to the deception imposed on us by the Local Authority. This was wrong, we said. This was not what we wanted done, nor was it according to the money that had been allocated to us.

The intransigence of the municipal officials hit us in the face like a bucket of cold water. Suddenly their tone changed. They accused us of instigating "the people". What they did not realise was that they were referring to the very people who had indicated through meetings that those schools would be boycotted until the matter was put right.

That was one of the things in 1985, which caused me to be detained. It was an issue on which representatives of the people had reached agreement with their Local Authority, yet it was on this very issue that officials of the Local Authority had turned tail. We had planned together with them but when the money had to be produced they did a somersault because they begrudged the money needed to uplift the standards of the Duncan Village people.

Another thing, which made them think I was a deeply involved activist, was that in my family almost everyone was an office-bearer on some little committee or other. Moreover, one of my five sons was in exile.

What I am most committed to in fact is the YWCA. Consequently young people tend to collect in my house. We regularly organise plays and other forms of entertainment, including beauty competitions. The constant presence of young people around me made the B.O.S.S. (Bureau of State Security) feel that I was an organiser for Umkhonti We Sizwe.

Unfortunately for me, my boy who left was in fact deeply involved in that line, something I was not informed of at that time. But I think they associated me with his involvement.

EDITOR'S NOTE

I should like to weave into this story, aspects of the detention of a British nurse – Doreen Norris – who spent a week behind bars after she refused to pay a fine for her participation in a protest against nuclear weapons. (Nursing Times: 5 August, Volume 83, No. 31,1987) The British prison officers reminded Doreen of the ward sisters during her training as a nurse. She was asked by a matronly wardress in the women's cells why a respectable person of her age was in that situation?. Her reply was: "I am a Christian and think it is very wrong to spend millions of pounds on weapons of destruction when people in the world are starving, sick and disabled.

The wardress is reported to have responded kindly. "*She listened to what I was saying*", said Doreen Norris.

CONSTANCE CONTINUES

I think these South African prison custodians learned a lot from us because we were a group who where not too badly educated while they had their heads buried in the sand. Every now and then, using the security guard as up-front man, we had to tell these people who we were and what we were saying through our organisations.

The domestic conditions into which we were hurled were totally appalling. One could imagine farmhands giving pigs a better deal. I was particularly perturbed to see that women are given a cold floor to sleep on. Is this how a civilised country treats its women? I felt sure that this was not how things ought to have been. And for that matter, for detainees to be given ragged, dirty blankets, I think that was not called for.

To me, when you are detained, you are taken away from your family, deprived of the opportunity to carry out your life tasks. I don't think that the treatment that you get in prison should be so utterly hurtful because you are being hurt already by staying there.

The diet was shockingly poor at first. At home our pets fare better. We hammered complaints at their door with woodpecker persistence until eventually it improved somewhat.

EDITOR'S NOTE

We return to Doreen Norris to discover what conditions were like for her.

LAHLEKILE

"I was taken into the prison. The doors were very firmly locked behind me. I was asked to undress and my belongings were taken from me and listed. I was given a prison dressing gown and all my clothes were taken away to be searched. I was then asked to go with a prison officer for a search. The dressing gown was removed and I stood naked; just me and my skin. Then I had a hot bath and afterwards was taken to another room to await a medical. By this time I had the dressing gown on again and felt more comfortable.

A very pleasant West Indian nurse took my medical history and I was beginning to feel much more relaxed. Some of my belongings were then returned … (she lists what she could or could not keep)….

I was taken to the reception wing and shown my room. I shared with three other women… I sat on my bed, thinking. The mattress was rock hard and there was only one pillow. There was a washbasin in the room, and a flush lavatory. Hooray, no slopping out. All in all the room was comfortable and warm.

At seven, the hatch in the door was opened and we were given rock cakes and a plastic mug of tea for our supper. I remember lying on my bed thinking. "I have a week of this". I fell asleep, my first day over.

At about seven the next morning the hatch opened again, someone wished us "good morning" and told us that breakfast was at 8am. I chatted with my fellow-prisoners who told me what to expect during the day. At 8am we filed outside and all the prisoners on the wing were taken to the dining room. Breakfast consisted of porridge, bread and marmalade and tea….

We had 15 minutes to eat before being taken back to our rooms and locked in.

At about 9am we were all taken to the exercise yard for half an hour. Before leaving the wing we were searched. The exercise area was surrounded by seats. Or we could spend our time walking round and round. Prison officers flanked the area from all sides.

Lunch was at 11:30am and "tea" at 3:30pm; these consisted of three cooked courses each. There was very little protein. Supper at 7pm was always served in the rooms. After tea, if the staff ratio allowed, we had a creation period. This meant we could mix freely with other prisoners on the wing or watch television if we wished.

One evening we were taken to the gymnasium to watch a volleyball match between the prisoners' team and the "eyes", the prison officers' team. The prisoners really enjoyed it and we all cheered when our team scored.

On the day after our arrival, it is the routine to be taken to see the assistant governor. She told me I would be released after five days, with good behaviour. I was informed of my rights and then I was told I must not tattoo myself during my stay in prison. She remarked that she realised I was in prison because of my principles. I found her attitude firm but reasonable.

One morning the hatch door opened and a loud voice said, "Norris for the special clinic." My immediate reaction was, no way, but then I thought of it as a way of getting out of the room for half an hour, so I went.

LAHLEKILE

On arrival a pleasant doctor told me that it was routine procedure to offer their facilities to all prisoners. I had to refuse his offer of a cancer smear as I have no cervix. This made him look down at my card. He saw I was only in for seven days and decided that perhaps their facilities would not benefit me. I heaved a sigh of relief, thanked him for his offer, bade him good morning, and beat a hasty retreat from his consulting room.

All in all I enjoyed my stay in Holloway. I found the prisoners interesting and lively... The prison officers were firm, but reasonable. They reminded me of the ward sisters when I trained as a nurse...

Because of my prison sentence my name has been removed from the register of the British Nursing Association. I was on their register for 35 years. This has upset me far more than going to prison, but I shall continue to protest against nuclear weapons, whatever the cost."

CONSTANCE TAKES UP HER STORY

The detention without trial was the worst experience of my life. There was a time when I was alone in a single cell. The toilet and everything else was crammed into the confined space. I lived on the ground like a bush animal, without seeing a human being for forty hours or more. It was a most horrible experience for me, with my ageing body and the great anxiety over the separation from my family, not to mention my dignity as a nurse and as a woman. For countless hours I would lie there rudderless and fractious.

Often it seemed as if the whole little cell crumbled or crushed towards me. There was the uncanny feeling of being squashed, like the crunching of a cockroach under a big boot, in as much as ever since I came out of detention I can't get into a lift alone. I always have that feeling of being brutally transformed into a small, insignificant object whose life is being snuffed out.

Another thing, which affected me while I was in detention, was forgetfulness. There was a time when my daughter brought my two precious grandchildren to visit but I was mortified to find that I had forgotten their names. It was an atrocious sensation trying to remember their names and it worried my daughter to see me thus afflicted. She realised that something was happening to her mother. Her complaints fell on deaf ears. We're not concerned with all this, their complicit smiles said.

Perhaps the worst experience of all was the gradual, then severe, then total occurrence of alopecia (loss of hair).

This degrading condition worsened when a purulent sore erupted on my scalp. Added to that an unsightly rash appeared all over my skin, which I could not recognise despite being a nurse. It spread with terrifying speed across my body. I have no doubt in my mind that the invading bacteria emanated from the dirty blankets. It was a happening, which made my stomach lurch.

The sore on my head did not resemble ringworm. I simply cannot put a name to it, but the pain it caused was insupportable.

My daughter was extremely perturbed and approached an outside doctor about my condition. He pulled some strings and treated me blind from the outside. But it was terribly debilitating and very itchy. I could not remember ever having felt so uncomfortable in all my life.

At other times I shared a cell with 33 other women. We had one shower to share between the lot. So when I needed desperately to reach water to wash the itchy head, this was only possible if it happened to be my turn. One could be swept by tears and yet not give way to them.

Similarly, it was a feat of endurance to stand in an endless queue in order to get under that shower to wash your crusty body. At such times personal unhappiness ran fathoms deep. To add insult to injury, privacy was a pipe dream.

You know, when you sit and think about such things, it raises formidable resentments because the people who make the rules, they never go and see what is happening and they have never been detained themselves. They know nothing of what is happening on the ground. Somehow the iniquities that exist will have to be rectified. If things could change in South Africa, I think people should be given an opportunity to plan for the future of state custody and it should be people who have experience of what is going on in every area of the Prisons Department.

I think that the South African Government should take a long, hard look into the treatment of detainees. There is so much that needs to be put right. Not the least of it is for prison employees to be able to differentiate between criminals and detainees.

At any rate we had to complain every day. This continual nag was the only way we could elicit a response.

The women warders were utterly ignorant and uncaring. Their thinking seemed devoid of any bit of refinement. They simply made the condescending assumption that we were common criminals.

Another terrible ill-health condition I suffered under the State's roof was that of persistent, intractable headaches. One time when such a terrible headache occurred I called for something to relieve it. I am allergic to aspirin and being a nurse, I had to tell them what I needed because of the allergy.

However, you are being undermined when you are behind bars, no matter how educated you are. It seems to them that when you go there, you leave your mind behind at your house.

I was forced to take something that made me very sick and in the end I made a statement about the treatment I got to the security officers. In the end it came to the position that people should be geared according to what they are. New rules were spilled out to defuse the clash of wills: nurses should be recognised as such and should not be forced to take things that they know are not beneficial to them. This eased a little the suffocating weight of white power.

INTERROGATION

This was more of an energy-sapping procedure than a painful one for me. Every now and again I was made to sit at Cambridge from 9am to 4pm.

The questions they asked over and over were:

WHEN DID YOU JOIN THE A.N.C.?
WHOM DID YOU RECRUIT?
WHY DID YOU INSTIGATE PEOPLE NOT TO PAY RENT?
WHY DO YOU ALWAYS HAVE YOUTH IN YOUR HOUSE?

I found the questions irritating, annoying, maddening, but I managed neither to fall into their trap nor to back down.

What I noticed was that the white security men were not overtly rude to me. They may have squinted from under their pale eyelashes or over the tops of tinted glasses, but they were not rude. I suspect that their unease at having to interact with a professional black woman ran very deep. What they did instead was to let the black security men be rude. These willing "serfs" shouted at me with hostility. Such scenes bordered on farce. I bridled at their bigotry, raked out my own cultural chauvinism as a defence mechanism and sprayed them with verbal venom:

"It is clear to me that you are not security people, you are nothing but tea boys or messengers, to talk so badly to us who are your people. Whenever we talk to these white people they at least listen and talk to us, but you call us names and are abusive. Your behaviour is unacceptable. Show some respect please, to women old enough to be your mothers."

All in all they were interrogating us on a regular basis up to the day, a year later, when I was released.

Before I left the prison they took me to be seen by a doctor. This was routine procedure. Then I was taken to another doctor because they felt that I might create problems for them when I got out and revealed the truth about my illnesses acquired while in their charge. That seemed to touch a live nerve in them.

At last the time came for me to go home. They said, "Here is 50c; now you may go home." I drew myself up to my full height, looked them in the eye and said: "I'll never go to a bus stop from here. You will take me and put me right in front of my house where you took me. It brought up an argument but in the end they capitulated to the fragile encounter with black female resistance. I was taken to my house, unlike every other "swallow" that is made to fly home on 50c.

GHALIMA

My career ended rather suddenly due to the capricious cruelty of a new supervisor who was an oxymoron of a person, doubtless of right-wing persuasion. Having been a matron for more years than I care to remember, my attitude was that of one who knew her duties and had no need to be reminded of them by anyone.

It was far from easy to work under direct white supervision all of a sudden, moreover under a person who loved to show an iron chin from day to day. She changed the functional structure in such a manner that we, as experienced matrons, were no longer able to run our wards without her express approval. Many of us were naturally repelled by her medievalism, which had us perpetually stung by reproof.

I'm not really political in outlook but at the back of my mind the suspicion grew that we ought not to go along with this. It would be as though we were willing to set up the machinery once again for formalised subservience, this when we are about to close the century. And who would be left to dismantle it again? None other than the young nurses of today. I was privately appalled.

My last days at Somerset were spent in an atmosphere of bleakness, resignation and despair. When the rationalisation process began, many of us eagerly seized the early retirement package and ran so fast you could not see us for the dust. There is hardly a single coloured matron left at Somerset these days, nothing to show the path of history, which they had pioneered for nursing. It was the boot of the oppressive Afrikaner, which had flattened us.

CONSTANCE

Difficulties in nursing began when I commenced duty at Frere Hospital in East London. Coming from the background of "Cora" and "Bara" to a mixed environment, which catered to different racial groups within the space of one hospital; well it was as though one had leaped into a snake - pit. The glaring black-white inequalities coiled itself around one's psyche like a deadly python, snuffing out every particle of happiness which nursing had provided on the Reef.

What was extremely embarrassing was to see that even if you were a senior nurse and a very experienced one at that, a white nurse of lower rank could come along and you would have to take orders from her. I deplored that aspect of professional life. It seemed that our people were inclined to bow to whites and inevitably I became drawn into this sick situation. You joined the troop because you needed the job but day-by-day you suffered the embarrassment of the slave to the master, hidden under rank differences. By unspoken consent black nurses laboured in silence. They avoided articulation of each day's tumultuous insults. By conspiratorial silence we hung on to the delicate thread of our employment.

Despite my apparent collaboration, the thread snapped for me when I was abruptly requested one day to hand in my resignation.

"I want you to terminate your duties at the end of the month." So stated Miss Gleaves (now late) who was the chief matron at the time. My eyes must surely have dilated with shock when I asked, "Why matron?" I can still hear the pitch and cadence of her voice when she replied curtly, "Because you have children. Go home and look after your children."

Naturally I was devastated. Yes, I was married and the children were a natural corollary to that, twins amongst them, but I needed the job. This was not only to supplement my husband's salary as a postal officer but to practice. So I had to write the letter of resignation, something which still raises my bile.

LAHLEKILE

I'm sorry that Matron Gleaves is not alive, because I am talking about her when she is not here. I truly dislike seeing one of the Frere buildings named after her because of what she did to me. She caused me to believe that the nursing world that we had been so excited about was somewhat of a flop.

It was no consolation later to discover - via the grapevine - that Miss Gleaves had wanted my post for someone else. Her action was a great put-down to me and it almost took apart the delicate fabric of my self-esteem.

Though the idea of having to stay home to look after my family may have sounded noble, my questioning mind brought the realisation that nursing administrators put out truths conveniently as they chose to see them. So although it was hurtful and unpleasant, I had to leave.

I secured a post at Lloyd's Clinic, under the East London Municipality, where I was orientated by a very strict sister. After coming through the waters of her baptism I acquired a positive reputation and soon ran the child health service on oiled wheels because of the excellent guidelines from her.

Overall it was lovely working in a community setting but as the years rolled on and my involvement in the political struggle became overt, I lost favour with the municipal nurse administrators who naturally preferred the status quo while ignoring the conditions that blacks were living under.

Things became infinitely worse under an Afrikaner who was brought in during my last years of duty. This person could have had right-wing affiliation because she exercised her authority over us in a most oppressive manner. Any of us who vented opinion in the work situation where easily put down by her. She made no attempt to hide her feelings in meetings and our suggestions were ill received. At planning level she would not allow active participation from us.

One distinctive feature of the whites in-charge was that reprimands could fall off their lips as easily as water from a leaking tap. In this they showed no remorse that they were dealing the adults who were entitled to being treated with respect.

This supervisor's attitude definitely affected me. I felt that my experience was important for practice, yet it was being effectively ignored, due to my involvement in the struggle. The climax of my activism was of course my detention without trial. After my release I experienced a major professional snub. The clock had barely stuck twelve to usher in my 60th birthday, when this diligent racist supervisor [who had no qualification to be a nursing service manager but earned the salary of one] effected my retirement with unseemly haste.

The fact that this oppressive person has since emigrated to America does not soften her deeds against myself and other colleagues. She promoted people without tertiary education to senior posts, overlooking those who had it, and the East London Municipality allowed this glaring abuse of power.

LAHLEKILE

NOMPUCUKO

I began training again at Frere Hospital under two capable sister tutors, Miss Dyani and Mrs. Njikilane. Many of us scored honours under them. I enjoyed medical-wards particularly mother-and-baby care and requested the maternity section on my application for a professional nurse's post. I was not to know then that my career would become tainted by one devastating occurrence, which filled my days with hurt.

It happened during a time when I was in-charge of the nursery and a baby died after being given a milk infusion by mistake. That was a most terrible thing. It was put up by a nurse who was doing her very last day of training, with the final exam already behind her. She had been a brilliant, swift and decisive student, one who had won our trust. Unfortunately, on this day she made a mistake when she administered milk intravenously into the drip already in place, instead of nasally. Since I was the sister-in-charge who had given her the instruction for the nasal feed I had to appear in court.

The case sizzled at first then dragged on for two then for three years during which time the legal net was woven ever more tightly around our heads. I had to prove that the nurse had been correctly instructed and that she had defaulted in the incorrect execution of that instruction.

At one time the girl's mother confronted me outside the court building. She subjected me to a devastating remark that the doctor and I were out to put her child in the wrong. The mother's motive was understandable but her remark set my nerves on edge. It plunged me into deeper depths of despair. The mother had procured legal assistance for her daughter in the hope that the blame could be made to stick at my door. The girl had put forward a version that could not easily comprise her.

Day by day the tension increased. Inside me it moved like a coil towards breaking point. Then at last came the outcome - the nurse was held responsible for "her own act of commission." The absolute truth was that the intravenous drip had already been in place when she was instructed by me to prepare the naso-gastric feed. What she had done was not to prepare the naso-gastric feed but to put the milk through the intravenous drip instead.

I cannot recall the sentence handed out, so great was the emotion that overwhelmed me but I believe that it was not heavy in terms of a jail sentence. In any event my own relief was buried beneath a blanketing weight of depression. As the sister-in charge I could not escape a moral responsibility. The case has left emotional scars which time cannot erase.

Other difficulties occurred but none that I could not manage, none that made me feel driven to give up nursing. There was a racial element, which left wounds of course, but gradually a shift has taken place, hardly discernable but it is there. With hindsight many incidents in the past now appear as amusing... For instance I recently visited someone in an Old Age Home. While there I passed an old white lady who was being assisted into a car. I recognised her as having been one of the housekeepers at Frere so I walked up to her with a friendly greeting.

We had worked together during a time at Frere when all I could secure was a housekeeper's job. At that time I was already doubly qualified in nursing. Those were the years when whites had to oversee blacks because the deep-cutting reality was that whites had always to be in-charge through the invisible "superiority". When I greeted the old housekeeper a shaft of amusement swept through me at my recollections of the past. By her greeting I could see that if this old lady ever had a conscience it could not have pierced too deep.

PULANE

My most memorable patient was Sonnyboy who was a paraplegic adult confined to bed because of complications with bedsores. He could not lie on his back for long so we had constantly to change his position from time to time.

When I think of Sonnyboy I remember how proud and high-minded he had been. It seemed possible that he might have been a dignitary in his time, crushed thoroughly by a tragic accident.

Sonnyboy was intensely domineering to the point that we junior nurses squawked and flapped around him. Actually I realise with hindsight that he was post-modern and deconstructive, the latter attitude because of his situation. No one could change his mind about anything he did not want done to him. He could hold a junior at his bedside for an hour or more, just to feed a burning cigarette to him whenever he had the urge to smoke.

Feeding him was an endless bore. We trembled in fear of this patient and he took advantage of his hold over us. We'd stand there, emotions fired up, feeding him for an hour, depending on how many interruptions occurred. Like a king on his dais his lordship would pay attention to whatever required his innocuous attention regardless of the captive junior armed with spoon and plate, standing dumb with willingness to serve.

In this modern era I have "de ja vu" when I think of Sonnyboy, that somehow I'd like for him to be transported back to this wonderful time of physiotherapists, social workers, occupational therapists, television, computers, you name it. How clearly can old approaches be remembered in the light of new conditions. We had none of the specialists neither the commodities yet we glided into the various roles with the ease of chameleons.

An enjoyable experience occurred at the time of the 1978 floods when all our carefully organised routine came unglued. Those of us who travelled together were the first to arrive at the hospital, first to get caught up in the floods during our routine. Water was flowing in at all ends so that closing the doors had no effect. The main kitchen was centrally situated which placed it out of reach. Linen was used to mop the floors.

In the aftermath we were amused to recall some of the incidents such as the sight of our dignified matron taking up the stance of a traffic officer on point duty. She had to direct our energies into a coherent modus operandi. Whatever difficulties we encountered were referred to her - "Matron we need this, we want that…" She fielded all the requests with seeming imperturbability, hair dripping wet and soft as duck-down.

LAHLEKILE

At one time she was soaked to the skin and began to peel of her clothes while we jumped around to form a human screen around her. She was sublimely unaware of the eager faces around her, thrumming with curiosity and anticipation, however she managed to slip into a theatre gown with impeccable dignity.

For all of us that flood was a first experience of its kind. When it was over we conducted workshops to strategise for future potential eventualities. With hindsight it was an experience that provided mirth by the bucketful, something often lacking in our serious lives.

Another crisis I experienced was when I administered pethidene to a wrong patient. It happened during a crucial time of bed shortages when one labour ward only had four beds but 21 patients. The manpower too was scarce as hen's teeth.

We were delivering cases in the townships, locally as well as further afield in the Eastern Cape. The Dora Nginza had not yet established maternity services. Our hospital averaged 900 cases per month.

On that fateful day I was up and running. Mrs. Peter was exceptionally busy too, so when I saw the doctors trooping in I offered to relieve her for their rounds. It was a day when everyone and everything rushed at you with rare intensity.

To my horror I gave the pethidene to the wrong patient. As luck would have it, it was Dr. Agnew's patient and he did not have the sweetest of temperaments. Two of us had checked the drug of course, but still it was administered to the wrong consumer.

I reported the error to Mrs. Peter the very second that I discovered it. She then reported the matter to Miss Fitchat, the matron of maternity while I personally broke the news to the doctor. He regarded me very attentively with impeccable self-control.

What was feared most was a complication on the baby; if this did not happen then there would not be a problem. In the end there were no complications. Everything went off very well. We had to appear before Mrs. Brussels, the chief matron, who reprimanded us (myself and the nurse-colleague) who had checked with me. Mrs. Brussels spoke in a calm and measured manner. After that the episode was placed on the backburner.

Another crisis occurred when I was supervising the pueperium ward where we were nursing up to a hundred patients at one time. We had to place mattresses on the floor but there were relatives who could not hide their shudders of revulsion at seeing wives, daughters and girlfriends on the floor and truly it was horrible. Tension mounted by the moment.

As a consequence we took a deep, steadying breath and decided to double them up on the beds. This caused a terrible flame of public anger to leap out, for now the patients did not know who they were sleeping with and they naturally disliked sharing space with strangers, most particularly with other cultures and races. Under such putrid physical conditions we had to deliver nursing care while dealing with closed rebellion from the staff.

In desperation we decided to put them together in terms of race/ethnicity - coloureds with coloureds, and so on. It came as no surprise when the patients recoiled from this arrangement too. There was a high level of dissatisfaction; every movement by one person caused the other person's nerves to sizzle. There was in addition a very definite degree of confusion.

So much so, that a patient from an outlying area called Green Bushes was discharged at the same time as a local resident. Tense like a coiled spring - due to the above circumstances of overcrowding in the ward - the Green Bushes mother left the premises with the wrong baby.

Fortunately her error was discovered within a short period during which time I had the awesome responsibility to sort it out by telephone, something I did as a supreme act of faith, hope and trust. In two shakes of a duck's tail, the farmwoman was back. Both babies still carried their name - tags; the exchange was made and the crisis averted. I experienced that unbelievable thump of relief that the case was so speedily resolved that it did not merit the attention on the authorities higher up.

NOZIZIWE

A nursing crisis, which I had to face, was a case of a circumcision gone horribly wrong. This child had ploughed through mud and rain all the way from his village across the Tsomo River armed with the requisition blanket. What went wrong was that the appointed "male nurse" who was suppose to have looked after them, covering their wounded area with special river leaves, had failed to turn up, consequently some of the boys had septic wounds in the area of circumcision.

All through the commotion of the admission procedure the thought entered my mind that no worse could surely happen than this, to a young person on the threshold of reproductive maturity with every man's pounding eagerness to prove his virility?

The doctor in charge of the case then began to put out feelers for a "special" nurse, one who would not only be capable of tender care but who could be trusted to keep everything in the greatest confidence. I was chosen and I see this as a singular achievement.

They showed me how to clean and dress the wound, which was raw, and having unstoppable ooze. The entire area was noisy - malodorous - with veins in the groin bulging like coiled snakes. The penis resembled a tattered rag. I had to clean this wretched, puny, shrivelled little thing while my heart leaped out to the will-o'-the-wisp boy-man. Wonderfully he recovered. Today he lives and works in Cape Town and never fails to look me up whenever he visits the Eastern Cape, at one time to show off his new bride.

If I could change things it would be in the area of discrimination against patients by the nursing fraternity. I work in a maternity section and though each patient naturally receives the best care in the labour ward because of the unique situation there, a different ethic prevails in the medical and surgical wards.

Professional nurses have a tendency of making a fuss of people they know, especially if these are relatives of themselves or colleagues. Conversely the disadvantaged patients are treated as though they come from the ragged edge of the universe.

LAHLEKILE

I pity the poor neglected patients who bear witness to staff members coming from all over the hospital to surround the bed of a "special" patient. There they stand bubbling their way through social conversation while the less fortunate lie as a captive audience, listening to how wonderful the other person's baby is. That must surely be a wounding experience.

If I could turn this attitude around, nursing would become a wonderful profession. After all, you are a nurse to the patients, not to a particular patient. There should be no social status, so I say let us stop classifying people.

MAUDE

I trained at Somerset Hospital before the advent of antibiotics and the development of medical technology. Today's treatment is sheer luxury for health professionals, compared with those barren days of the mid-century. The length of training was 3 1/2 years for general and 1 1/2 years of midwifery. These years moved with lightning swiftness because we were too fatigued to count time.

My most memorable patient? Well, there were two men lying side by side in the medical ward. They reminded me of the biblical character Lazarus - the poor beggar - and the rich man, who in this case was clad in silks and had an attitude to go with it.

When he deigned to speak to anyone his tone was as cool as the drip of ice. The "poor" man lay in the bed next to him but was effectively cold-shouldered by having a rigid back turned to him at all times. The "poor" man's only response to this snub was a bleak gleam of astonishment from the sable darkness of his eyes.

The privileged man had a volatile personality that was difficult for us to cope with. He could inflame or incite us by being deliberately or provocatively rude. When one performed a task for his comfort he would reproach one furiously with ingratitude.

He used to swear at his family, the priest and the church groups, reacting to the latter as though they had laid a blight on his spirit. It was exceedingly difficult to get close to him and to offer any comfort, yet he was in the terminal stage of his illness. I remarked to my colleagues, "I hope that this man dies when we are not on duty because I sense that he is evil". It was an impassive feeling but now that I am away from it, it can still shake the nervous system.

Poor "Lazarus" on the other hand, was a wretched, puny, humble patient with such a tremendously generous spirit that he gave and received a great deal of warmth. The memory of the contrast between the two is deeply engraved on my mind.

Nursing in Barkley West [a rural area] brought one up against enormous difficulties, so much so, that I resigned because of practice modes that I found intolerable. Firstly there was the racial discrimination. The straw that broke the camel's back was the shocking treatment that the white nurses meted out to the black patients. That went against the grain.

LAHLEKILE

For example a doctor would prescribe Tetrex but the white nurses would come along and change the prescription to Sulphadiazine, which was cheaper. This unethical and illegal practice went on without any intervention from above. One had to grit one's teeth because life goes on no matter what. In the light of hindsight I can see that I belonged to a generation of nurses who obstinately clung to a dream. We needed to liberate ourselves from the poverty at home and nursing seemed to be a gateway to a brighter future. So we accepted the feeling of self-respect and the idea of progress in exchange for a life'- sentence of hard labour, deprivation and racial cruelty, all this in silence.

Another thing that posed a difficulty for me was the fact that frail-aged blacks had to be awakened and washed at four am, which troubled me greatly. I found this so very cruel, waking people up and exposing them to the cold and pre-dawn darkness. The reason given was because of shortage of staff. I have raised the issue time and again in an attempt to turn around the tacit invincibility of the powers-that-be. Eventually the problem came to be addressed due to my persistence. Frail-aged patients are now being attended to when the day-staff come on duty.

The other thing that I found hard to swallow was the racial discrimination against black professional nurses. Across this scenario I think the salary discrimination was the worst aspect. On the whole it is true to state that a white assistant nurse was paid better and treated with higher regard.

Around 1966 I transferred to the Red Cross Hospital in Cape Town, after which I went over into the community health field. This last change opened up a palpitating vista with many rich experiences but there was a major obstacle in the way. There were thugs roaming the streets looking for confrontations with all and sundry. At that time they seemed to have lost respect for the whole of society.

I was engaged in the Family Planning service so we travelled from point to point and met a great diversity of people and groups. Our fears rose with the discovery that our uniform was no longer a protective shield. What most marked the "skollies" was their cruel, mindless spirit of mischief. There was something indescribably sadistic in their persecution of innocent people. Fortunately we were always two in the official vehicle or the daily brutality of the skollies might have harmed us or upset our reason. A happy sidekick of community work was that we often were in the industrial setting so we had access to the factory bargains that Cape Town is famous for.

What I enjoyed most of all was to be trusted and put in charge of a ward. I was proud as a pouter pigeon when I became a senior nurse on the ward and the doctor asked, "who is in charge?" I would step forward, heart swelling with pride, eager to demonstrate cooperation, creativity and initiative. I still view myself as having achieved excellence in hands-on nursing care.

CALABASH

Going far back in time to my own training I remember a minor crisis, which had hit me on the very first day. I had been assigned the task of cleaning sputum mugs, a task so unpleasant that one's nose twitched in constant revulsion. This was how blue juniors fresh from home were required to handle raw infection, ostensibly to desensitise them to Tuberculosis.

The fancy taps played games with me in this strange place called a "sluice room". When I opened the first tap the water shot up in my face and nose causing me to cough, splutter and gasp. I opened the second one keeping clear of the first but rivulets of water again showered me till I was soaked to the skin. One of the patients bounded in to rescue me.

There is a reason why I could never forget that first day. I wore silk black stockings, an incredibly important event, not only for my gawky adolescence but also for not having had cover for the legs and feet during the years of growing up. By teatime that day the silk stockings were hanging in shreds while I snivelled into my tea.

The second crisis I remember well is the flood of 1968. It happened on a Sunday morning. At first I was insulated by the hospital environment, not knowing of the flood that had burst upon Port Elizabeth without warning. It was only when I left my office to go to tea that I became aware of the disaster.

Upon my return from tea everything was dark due to a power failure. I was in charge of the Paediatric section with babies in incubators and some on oxygen, others crying incessantly. The Burns Unit had patients and I became increasingly distraught especially when some nurses were struck by lightening. A mood of unspeakable misery hung over us. The flood was hitting the premises with a vengeance. Steadying myself with one hand against a wall I slowly marshalled my wits and strength, firstly to deal with the sobbing nurses. I had to fight back a sense of suffocation.

As soon as the nurses were calm my thoughts gravitated towards the safety of the patients. Swiftly I led the nurses into a pattern of action. One dilemma was whether or not we should open the windows or switch off the oxygen, or what? The cerebrum sprang into gear while apprehension arose in the breast. With thumping heart I switched off the air conditioner and opened the windows. Speechless with relief I realised there was no fire. The full magnitude of what was happening struck me with the force of a physical blow. All of Port Elizabeth was flooded and flushed. One butcher's had all its meat out in the street looking as though it had been smitten by a thunderbolt.

One of the enjoyable experiences happened on that day that I was promoted to "sister". I pranced about excitedly; it had taken so long. In 1954 after completing my training I had been a spirited, self-possessed, competent person, yet I only got promoted in 1965. This kind of suppression exposes the cracks and wrinkles in South African nursing. We were kept "staff-nursing" for years while promotion was allowed to be the domain of white nurses. It was an easy option for them while it percolated our way very slowly. We took these hurts quietly.

Another source of enjoyment was to see a patient who had come in very ill, improving to the point where he could grasp the reigns of his own life once again. If you had a direct hand in his care there was an extra uplift of heart when he went home.

LAHLEKILE

I remember a patient who had undergone an Oesophagectomy and Mr. Thatchel had put a Naso-gastric tube in place. On the second day I observed that there was no drainage and that the abdomen was enlarging. On my own initiative I took out the tube and replaced it. I was working with a white colleague, one of those whose promotion had been jarringly sudden. She was less qualified than I was and we were like two bears that could not get along in one den.

When she saw what I had done she proceeded to harangue me and went as far reporting me to the surgeon who immediately realised that I had adroitly saved the patient much discomfort. After my intervention there was blood drainage and the abdomen had subsided nicely yet there I was, standing by anxiously awaiting the complications that she was predicting with malicious certainty. However the patient did not complicate at all. He was discharged happy and well.

LINDA

A crisis situation began to build up at the time of the 1976 riots. We had to close down for a few days while management made decisions from which we were of course excluded. At that time the riots came as a shock, people were simply not prepared. It proved a harsh lesson for all of us.

During the mid-eighties when social unrest again reverberated through the townships things had vastly changed; you could detect aggression arising in the nurses, quite a change from the former nurse who never answered back.

Doreen Merle Foster

Irrespective of where they were situated the oppressed nurses became involved. It was a time when the arms of the state killed people with indifference. We had to run emergency outlets from our own homes, taking out bullets, stitching wounds. That is when the concept of primary health care (PHC) worked. However, we ran into a problem through lack of antibiotics, something that we could not prescribe.

They were GP's in the township who came to our rescue; they not only assisted us but became the source of antibiotics, which we were unable to lay our hands upon. We did our job as nurses in spite of the convulsions brewing around us, referring the major medical tasks to the doctors-of-the-people, who made a magnificent contribution.

I should like to recount an incident, which had me almost jerk out of control. It happened in 1991 when a white superior was brought into our situation. She appeared to me to be a member of the extreme right wing such as the AWB [Afrikaner Weerstandsbeweging (Resistance Movement)].

Upon our first encounter she asked whether I have a degree and how it came about that I landed a post as chief professional nurse, to which I replied facetiously, "Some are born great, others have greatness thrust upon them."

Each time I went to her office she would rake her eyes over me from the shoes upward. At first I felt intimidated and besieged but she could not lift the positive outlook I had about my work. Until one day when I forewarned her that I might require permission to extend my lunch hour a fraction since I had to go to the bank with a weighty problem concerning my son's stop-order.

As predicted I was held up and returned 15 minutes late. First she stared at me as though I were a two-headed calf, then she unleashed a storm over my head, which stopped just short of vituperation. Her attitude smacked slightly of megalomania. I actually experienced agony over her rudeness. From that time onwards our working relationship lay in tatters. She would pick up the phone and bark, "Go to such a place and do this or that."

We're talking 90's here.

Far worse, was that whenever I departed from my office to some point of work she would phone there before my arrival leaving cheeky messages – which downgraded me to my own people – that I was to phone immediately upon arrival to inform her as to why I had not been there when she called.

One such incident proved to be the final ignominy piled upon the many indignities I had to suffer.

Inevitably, I made my way to the most senior person-in-charge to enunciate clearly some very angry feelings, which were boiling up within. I told her that I was about to inform the head office of CPA [Cape Provincial Administration] that I intended resigning from my post because of this "AWB" woman standing sentinel over me.

Firstly, I said, the Family Planning service employs people, not political parties. The programme provides for all the people of South Africa not a particular race group.

Secondly, I also intended informing the head of CPA that I understood now why my people, the African people, were so very angry out there, if they had been exposed to people like *her* who traded on their white skins to badger blacks from their power positions. And thirdly, should this woman be here much longer I would walk out.

At the end of the day she and others like her, will be dealt with by all the little Winnie Mandelas who are tumbling through the gates of UWC (University of the Western Cape), highly-qualified and who will hound bigots like her out of office in seconds flat.

The senior person I was reporting to – obviously stranded in a cultural sandbag – had the grace to blush when I said to her, "You will never have a woman of my calibre and integrity working in and around the Western Cape. I shall not be unemployed for even one month. Right now, you have peace in the townships largely because of my efforts, and this is the way I am treated in this department?

That was the day when Linda was churning inside. I was a prowling tiger, angry enough to exorcise the horror of this particular form of oppression that had yoked us for decades.
I was confronting it head on. Whatever I forgot to say and remembered when I returned to my office would have me do an about-turn to confront her again, while breathing like a steam engine.

I would say, "Listen, phone the City Health Department and ask them who is this angry black woman facing you today? I have served them for 22 years; the files don't rot; they will retrieve them from the archives and you will then know whom you are dealing with. I'm not unscrupulous, when I look at a person I do not look at the colour of their skin."

Thus my thoughts jumped tracks as I deflected my anger. After a while that person left the service. She could not last because she was unable to change her attitude. Her departure barely caused a murmur and from me there was no olive branch; our paths had parted in anger. I said to her, "Thank you for having ill-treated me. In one way you have assisted me to make an important decision. I had other intentions but now I shall join the Pan Africanist Congress, if only for their slogan "One heart one bullet."

This tumbled out spontaneously. I have no doubt that my words shocked everyone, for the act of disclosure of political affiliation is for administration sensitive in the extreme, especially if it carried any whiff of organised resistance.

PART 3 - ACHIEVEMENTS & PROPOSALS FOR CHANGE

MID-CENTURY TRAINEES

CONTRIBUTORS TO THIS SECTION

1. Regina
2. Mekiwe
3. Nyameka
4. Gladys
5. Mary
6. Constance
7. Ghalima
8. Ntombizodwa
9. Calabash
10. Maude
11. Pulane
12. Nozizwe
13. Eugene
14. Linda
15. Nanziwe
16. Calabash
17. Chloë
18. Nompucuko

MEKIWE

My first priority for change would be remuneration. Across the entire century nurses have led lives filled with financial stress most especially of course the black nurses. Now that politicians are bending over backwards to erase the past this has got to be speedily altered.

Working conditions too. I'm thinking along the lines of an exchange system for nurses. I experienced such a scheme during my training in Durban. We were burdened by overseas nurses coming out to South Africa to broaden their experience. They circulated between King Edward, Mc Cords and Addington. It was our task as senior nurses to take charge of them though they had completed their training. They would say, "Oh we are so happy to have *you* as our mentor for now we can learn more comfortably from you; to us everything is new."

I am sure that if such schemes could be introduced here it would inspire South African nurses to greater performance heights. It might succeed in changing nut-hard attitudes. More importantly, it could pave the way for new models to be effected in nursing.

Finally there is the question of specialisation. We have orthopaedics and paediatrics opened up and I know someone currently engaged in a PHD for psychiatric nursing. We need to be more knowledgeable for the 21st century, more ready to teach and to fertilise the knowledge base through our diversity of academic prowess.

PULANE

Though it raises a blush there is quite a sheaf of achievements I can claim credit for. In the past it was a great difficulty for anyone to have to take charge of the labour ward. It takes a special kind of leader to be able to buffer her self against the dislocations embodied in this work.

When I was in charge of a labour ward one of my first endeavours was the empowerment of each and every sister as far as the running of that ward was concerned. I laid a foundation for any member of the trained staff to be able to rise to the challenge of running that ward, of taking charge.

Another innovation on an entirely different scale was the introduction of morning prayers. Now it happened that my daughter came to Dora Nginza to deliver and she mentioned to me in passing how in Mmabatu they would group themselves for the purpose of prayer.

I found the idea charming, strategic, definitely a tradition to imitate. I felt that there was a need to value this form of black religious and cultural expression.

The Pillar Nutritional Group was another innovation. Some of us had attended a most inspiring presentation on nutrition at the Baragwanath Hospital. The speaker was a Mr Gali. Upon our return we started a follow-up group with the blessing of Dr Freeman, our paediatrician. He was pleased that we intended following up malnutrition cases from hospital to home without reimbursement. It was regarded as a remarkable agenda, by all the doctors, nurses doing such valuable work without prescription or coercion.

One home remains unforgettable, if only for our efforts to clean the dirt. It was an urban environment where naked children, emaciated dogs and scrawny chickens scrabbled in filth. Inside the house there were clumps of debris rotting either there or outside in the burning sun. The mother worked away from home leaving Nokwanda the baby, with a small child who had to be at school at noon. She would be relieved by another sibling who came at 2pm. Mrs Orlayne (now chief nursing service manager) was my colleague, my friend, and my mentor. We brought detergents and things from home and scrubbed and swept with great determination.

To us, this vital corollary to our work in the hospital proved deeply satisfying. We were apparently used as an example to the Durban nurses who were told "Port Elizabeth nurses go the extra mile doing voluntary follow-up work after hours and over weekends."

After the 1986 riots when communities became senseless, we were suddenly viewed as alien beings. One lady, also engaged in volunteer work and belonging to the community, was stopped from handing out food parcels one day and was burned to death at that senseless time.

When that happened it was reason enough for us to abandon our project. The Pillar Nutritional Group had to shuffle out of the people's lives, the choice had to be made. Yet we loved our time with them enormously. The mother of the house described above had begun imperceptibly at first, to do for her self. By the time we left she was treading the path of cleanliness, which we had opened up.

As far as change is concerned, I think that mechanisms ought to be put in place for acknowledgement. This is a terribly emotive factor. People do things that are simply marvellous and they leave the profession without a single token of appreciation.

Mrs Ben-Mazwi's group was more unfortunate than ours for we at least received wrist watches to commemorate our dedicated service. This is a very specific quibble; one that I think bears closer scrutiny. Look at the sacrifices, which someone like Mrs Ben-Mazwi had made during her time. For example her name is practically synonymous with flood relief.

She overcame countless ups and downs, which would have diminished a lesser person. Yet all of her efforts came to nothing as far as acknowledgement is concerned, no cracking of Champaign bottles and I think it is a shame.

Now that I have gone on early retirement I wish to express my extreme dissatisfaction with the statutory bodies. There is nothing coming our way, quite besides speech making and hoopla, there is not even the words "Thank you" to give the heart a bound. It has caused a chronic and permanent pain.

To think that we assisted them all these years as shock absorbers between themselves and the students. We were the ones who blindly bound together the disparate operations – like white superiority, respect and loyalty – within the apartheid system of nursing into a cohesive whole. We did this in all innocence of course; political scales plastered over our minds' eye by nursing ethics and philosophies. At the end of the day they remained paternalistic to us while we earned the hatred of the students who were absolutely contemptuous of the notion that we subserved their cause by filling in the sandwich.

LAHLEKILE

Another crucial plank in nurse thinking, which begs change, is the age of retirement. It is ludicrous that the black nurse (unlike the white who all too soon becomes an pen-pusher) has to be so run off her feet that after the age of 60 she begins to hate everyone around her. That was my personal experience. You are then no longer able to give of your best to the patient.

Our requests to have the retirement age reduced were shot down in flames. This without any meritocracy, without any understanding of the pressures of what was going on in nursing. There was absolutely no interaction between us older nurses and the people serving on the statutory bodies who clung to their dominant management role. That was monstrously unfair. They ought to have gone far enough into understanding and analysing the resistance of current nurses to the status quo.

Nowadays the workflow is unpredictable. Whatever happens in nursing is governed by politics with the nurses themselves being kept in a state of being *a-political*, something that is no longer possible or desirable. My proposal is that retirement ought to be made optional from the age of 55 years.

What is terribly bad these days is the toyi-toying of nurses; having one's surname written up on placards to be downgraded as matrons; hearing them agitate for your removal from office. What I want to know is: do we deserve to be reduced to quivering wrecks by the withering inquisitions of the unions? None of us deserve that, not after 40 years of devoted service.

Furthermore, the secrecy with which our financial affairs are managed must be uncovered. Nothing is laid openly on the table - everything is a hidden agenda. It is of paramount importance that nursing administrators be made accountable. The current position is that when an administration clerk explains things to you it is not possible to trust what is being said, to eagerly gulp done everything at one big swallow.

When we left, we said we no longer cared (after countless explanations) if they gave us a mere snippet. If the few cents we were left with led to a tomorrow, when we'd have to go around picking up orange peels in the streets, that would be fine. All we needed when the early-retirement packages became available was to get the dust of the toyi-toying situation off our heels. After all, one's time is circumscribed.

The 90's is a time that is both dynamic and unstoppable. My colleagues and I have nothing but good wishes for today's progressive nurses who are opening the door to a new age in nursing. Their activism is inevitable and imminent. But we deserve our release; our time has passed.

I remember a case of triplets whom we had decided to place on our caseload. We were familiar with our townships where people lived in the most miserable conditions and were rapidly sinking in the social scale. We recognised the urgency with regard to the triplets.

So we followed them up for a year. Unfortunately the parents were of the unschooled variety. They were conditioned and not able to move outside that conditioning.

LAHLEKILE

After a year they removed the triplets to a rural area of the Transkei where we feared that a human tide of poverty would sweep over them. In fact one baby died, it was news that twisted an ache in the collective breast.

The house was simply beyond description. Mrs Orlayne was my colleague, my friend, mentor and strongest supporter in the project. (Mrs Orlayne is currently the senior nursing service manager of the Dora Nginza Hospital).

When this became established practice on the general and later the maternity side, both patients and staff expressed enjoyment for it.

In the community I was the chairman of the Pillar nutritional Group. It so happened that Mrs Mpondo (now late) accompanied me to the Baragwanath Hospital in the 660's where a Mr Gali gave a most inspiring presentation on nutrition. When we returned we decided to shift the induced boundaries of nurse-consciousness by starting a follow-up group, something, which took us into the domain of creative invention.

We informed firstly the paediatrician-in-charge (I've forgotten his name), then Dr Freeman who came after, that we intended to follow-up all the malnourished cases needing attention. That was regarded as a remarkable agenda, nurses doing their own thing without prescription or coercion.

NYAMEKA

As far as achievement is concerned, I've been preaching *RESPECT AND CARING* through the years, having felt insulated in a life that had no references other than the ethics of nursing. To change attitudes takes a long time but it can be done by persuasion and example.

In the theatre where vulnerability was plain, it was possible for me to chip away the arguments and disagreements, which sprang up over tiny practicalities. I encouraged the nursing staff to take cognisance of the idiosyncrasies of the different surgeons. That is what I imprinted on my subordinates; to work with the doctors not against them. Nowadays one cannot easily do that. Today they cheek the doctors and pile torments on us "golden oldies" calling us "ja-baas" people.

In no small measure I can claim credit for research. The area of my investigation was late coming at the hospital. When the nursing colleagues discovered this their expressive dark eyes recoiled with shock. They said, "Oh, so you're sitting here in your car watching us come late on duty?" A deep sigh swept through me at this misperception. And a very sad thought crossed my consciousness – will we ever have pedigree in nursing?

At a later stage I was approached by another colleague doing theatre technique. She had phoned for permission to come and see me "pertaining to the study you are doing." When she came I discovered that she wanted a toehold on my findings and on the details of the research method I had followed. Much later on the penny dropped at the hospital that what I was engaged in actually had tremendous worth, whereas before there was this hostile response causing one or two people to be gratuitously rude to me.

The research galvanised my mental energies and restored my focus. I used a generalisation method to unearth many problems causing late coming. As a result of this study I was able to recommend that the hospital establish a crèche nearby to address a yawning need, similarly the acquisition of a bus for nursing and non-nursing personnel. I have had word that they were cutting through the bureaucratic bush to set the ball rolling to percolate this idea into the stony heart of administration.

When it comes to change, money is the first thing, which springs to mind. Admittedly it goes against the grain since one does not like to think of remuneration in terms of a caring profession. But I say, give the nurses a decent package then we'd have sparkling nurses who will be relaxed and caring towards their patients. It would go a long way to reduce nursing's worst nightmare, nurses on the toyi-toying rampage demanding better pay.

Discrimination in salaries is another sore point. Look at the difference in hospital workloads. When whites talk about a ward, how many patients are they dealing with compared to us? The nurse-patient ratio is glaringly different. The ludicrous situation is common, that a 20-bed facility can have more (white) nurses than a 64-bed facility on the black side. Yet salaries are not adjusted accordingly. This is an issue over which the state needs to be confronted. It is simply incredulous that nurses are not better rewarded.

NANZIWE

During the decades of the practice years there were many difficulties, perhaps the most notable of these was the writing of progress reports. Those years the white matrons became energised when you presented black nurses in a poor light. If you did not bring nurses to the office to be scolded, then they gained the impression that you – as supervisor – were not doing your work properly. It was pure speculation of the lowest kind.

I once worked with a care-worn sister who worked in OPD for a very long time and then she was taken to the gynae ward where I was in charge. By this time everyone had trodden her down spitefully in their reports; the office had this indelible impression that this sister was useless but when I worked with her I found that the very opposite was true.

Mine must have been the first favourable report sent in because I was called to be questioned as to whether my version was a true picture. The matron's eyebrows were raised to the roof. I stood by my claim, ready to fly in the face of popular opinion. When that sister left Livingstone for St Mathews Hospital she was promoted with astounding velocity.

At one point in my career I decided to go to England for training in theatre technique. In South Africa the whites were jealously guarding this domain and I decided to challenge that.

I had no theatre experience whatsoever, having come from Livingstone where only white sisters worked in theatre with black staff-nurses to assist them. My first difficulty in England was language because it was simply not easy to follow their various accents.

I shall never forget the very first case on the slate. It was for a sex change op. Suddenly I was confronted with a major culture shock. It was the skin prep. That had brought it on. For my eyes to have fallen for the very first time on a white body – without the sky crashing down on me – well I realised in a daze what numbing effect apartheid had on the psyche. It took all of three months before white bodies ceased to be an oddity.

I kept on dropping bowls and things on the floor at the shock of the white bodies. Each time this happened the surgeons and nurse colleagues teased by saying, "Drums of Africa" It had the effect of tearing down my defences and rendering me a trifle foolish. After that I was fine, enjoying the year immensely.

Upon my return I was able to penetrate the hallowed portals of a South African operating theatre where whites ruled supreme. I was actually pressurised by a white matron, incredible as that might sound. She seemed to enter into a conspicuous rivalry with me. It was clear to me, fresh from England, that it would take a long time to change the hard hearts and closed minds of those South African whites that support the system. I was the first black sister who was allowed to work in theatre amongst five white sisters and a few black staff nurses. When I got there, there was one small change-room, which we shared. The white sisters had their own enormous office and were served tea from the kitchen while the staff nurses and I had to walk 10 minutes to reach the Nurses' Home where we had our tea. I decided to challenge this injustice.

This was the beginning of a lengthy struggle fighting for rights. I said, "I am also a sister and I want my share of tea and sandwiches. Furthermore I want my own office unless we can share one office. After countless fights that battle was won.

Another issue which rubbed me up the wrong way was that the staff nurses were not allowed to scrub; but they had to set all the trays just for the white sister to step up like a conductor about to wave the baton. I looked at the situation and then took it up with the authorities. I said, "If blacks can get out all the instruments and can set all the trays, why can't they scrub? At the end of the day this bastion of apartheid also came crashing down.

With eye surgery I decided to make it a test case for me. With a nonchalant suggestion "Let me do eyes today" I prepared to scrub. A Sister Thomas came along and asked what I thought I was doing? I replied, "I'm going to scrub for this case." Her lips distorted into a grimace when she asked insultingly, would I know what to do? I replied, "Well, I'm depending on the surgeon to ask for what he wants; it's as easy as all that."

One day my feathers were ruffled over off-duties that had been tampered with. A mistake had been made whereby 4 hours would have passed with no white supervision so she changed this crudely and hastily. I said to her, "I shall not accept these off-duties that you are making out now. Just because my skin is black you think that I cannot be in charge?" She deplored my stance, my extravagant language and leaped up the grievance ladder.

LAHLEKILE

In the chief matron's office once again the colour prejudice superseded a basic sense of justice. I said firmly, "If I cannot be trusted because of the colour of my skin then kindly take me out of theatre and put me back in the wards." Within a short span of time this route was in fact taken. There was nothing apocalyptic about *their* point of view.

When the Dora Nginza Hospital opened, giving the first-time chance to blacks to start a hospital from scratch, at last we came into our own. Mrs Peter (now late) and I were amongst 19 guinea pigs that were sent to Kalafong College in Pretoria (we were two blacks from each province) to do DNA (Diploma in Nursing Administration) I had ward Administration under my belt but Miss Brussels forced me to repeat the course. She said, "I'll never promote you unless you do it." Of course I leaped into the water. Who does not want promotion?

I have just remembered another enjoyable experience I'd like to share. One day I was confronted by a set of doctor's orders that was Greek to me, you know how awful their handwriting can be? Staring up at me in an ugly scrawl were the words G.O.K. or so we thought. In the end I had to phone the doctor concerned for an explanation. He came charging up to the ward from casualty (Dr Njongo is late now), looked at us pensively for a long moment while smoking his pipe and then he said explosively, "It's God-only-Knows because I don't."

I've had several achievements though one is loath to blow one's own trumpet. I received a certificate of appreciation from the Voluntary Aid Bureau of Port

Elizabeth in recognition of voluntary service for SANCA, signed by the mayor.

Then there was a certificate of recognition of meritorious service for community activities, something I am yet engaged in [at the time of writing]. The certificate was for outstanding service. To this day the restless spirit forever moves in me.

As far as change is concerned I belong to the old school of bedside nursing. My focus in teaching students has always been, "Do unto others what you have done for yourself." Just to bring home the point of a full wash, a clean mouth, of being comfortable along every inch of your person before you even eat. I say, "You did all these things, including a visit to the toilet did you not? That is all that we are asking here - do for the patients what you have done for yourself."

There is a very old colleague who worked in Dora Nginza's time during the 1920's. She is today quite decrepit, blind and paralysed. Bound to a wheelchair she is nevertheless quite lucid. Now look at her situation. She devoted her adult life to nursing countless patients but what nursing care is she getting today? I think a value for human life must be brought back.

All of us "golden-oldies" with our hypertensive conditions, have got this prayer in our hearts that when our times comes, that it be a quick stroke, then gone by God's hand. We should hate to fall into the hands of today's nurses. Look at the hospital environment. It is beyond dirty, absolutely filthy. So I say, back to basics.

LAHLEKILE

CALABASH

An achievement that I am proud of was my involvement with a group called the Pillar Nutritional Group.

This was a small organisation started by nurse colleagues to promote better nutritional practices amongst the poorer section of the New Brighton community. We entered the township homes to ferret out children who were malnourished and who had physical defects. It is difficult to imagine what would have become of them had they remained locked away.

Without being stiff-necked I claim credit for the success of my nursing education career. There was never a time when the mantle of tutor hung heavily upon my shoulders.Indeed when I first began teaching post-basic courses in paediatrics from 1986, my chest simply filled with excitement. When I retired this experience proved to have been the most enjoyable of all.

In my memory-arsenal of students – and these include pupil-nurses, diploma-nurses, 4-year students – there were those who, with large lustrous eyes, had received gold medals, distinctions, honours; of course there would be failures too, but I enjoyed the success of my students. With the state of nursing as it is today, I should not apportion any blame to myself for non-caring attitudes. I relish the knowledge that I had only given of my best.

An achievement of lesser glory occurred out of my sojourn in the wards when infection was rife. I was quite particular about the prevention of infection in paeds and insisted on the use of gowns and masks.

I actually researched the spread of infection caused by opening wounds for the surgeon's rounds. Translating this finding into a vision, I wrote a letter to the chief matron making a proposal. I stated, "Could we not have some cover, like sterilised draw-sheets, so that wounds could be lightly covered by this means instead of inviting every termite to feast until the surgeons arrive?" Eventually what we got were burns sheets with brown tags. It served the purpose and I was happy for that, although there was not even muted applause for this thing, which I had innovated.

I should prioritise for patient well being first. During the 1990 boycott my heart bled when I visited a friend of mine who had suffered a stroke. The visit brought me face to face with reality.

I found this very old lady naked on the bed, which had no sheets. She was drooling, with not a soul around to help her. I looked around and discovered that the entire ward was in a state of abysmal neglect. Meanwhile the nurses were toyi-toying outside; the thought made my head ache relentlessly.

I returned to the college and from there we rushed across to do our bit though we were too few to make much of an impact. We prepared food, fed children, helped to feed helpless patients, served meals to the others. Had we not come by they would have starved. I would definitely put the welfare of the patient before everything else.

Secondly the well-being of the nurses, who ought not to find themselves in a position where they need to go down so low as to neglect patients in their care. Today's nurses are provoked to the utmost and feel compelled to take such untoward action. Due to an unacceptable manpower shortage the nurses work like packhorses with poor remuneration and no recognition. This is a controversy that has mushroomed to a formidable extent.

Thirdly I propose incentives in nursing. Not only would incentives release a powerful energy, it could change the values too. The state could stick its nose in here. There is no logic in keeping it's nurses in low esteem and grinding poverty.

Lastly, good education cannot be over-emphasised. In my view anybody who has to handle a patient should have a good education. There should be no grading of nurses; we should all have one nursing education so that we can have a collective inordinate pride in our profession. If you look at the standard of education of the nurses out on strike you will see that it is mostly the subcategories that have never been upgraded in any way. This is terminal enslavement. There should be a consideration of the advancement of the nurse educationally and professionally.

I am therefore prioritising for a good educational background for nursing. Management philosophies should bow to the times. The future nurse must be well educated academically and professionally.

In the middle part of the century nurses had a minimum JC education yet expectations were high. My suggestion is that all persons applying for nursing are required to have passed matric so that the lower grade can be eliminated.

In conclusion I'd like to say that opportunities for advancement ought to be the same for all nurses irrespective of race or sex. There is an urgent need to cancel out the resentments and frustrations culminating in shoddy practice. Educators should produce nurses free from apathy of spirit who can be proud of their profession.

LINDA

Our service was doctor-oriented which carried a major problem to the nurse who consequently was not allowed to make decisions. Incredibly, it seemed a lesser evil for her to allow a patient to die rather than to practice beyond her scope, beyond their immutable set of rules.

In other words, between 1967 and 1980 you had to listen to another health care provider's aspirations without having the power to be creatively involved in your practice. This demonstrates to me a shocking paucity of utilisation of the nursing talent.

The entire problem in health delivery in this country began in the past when horses were put at the back of the cart. We have to view the community as a system. Now what we did was to take the nursing culture and base it in the hospital, far from the community, whereas, nursing should commence from the preventive and promotive perspective.

This mistake is the direct outcome of the Health Act of 1936, which was brought into being because of the 1918 flu epidemic. On a daily basis people were dying by the score so the health authorities got together to tackle the problem. That is how the hospital concept of health care emerged. Five decades later when the primary health care (PHC) concept evolved from the historical conference at Alma Ater in Russia, this was not accommodated in the South African Health Act. Today the oppressed majority is so besieged by hunger, want and misery; the pattern has become so familiar, that most nurses have become numb to the situation. It is the Health Act, which needs essentially to be revised.

There are, in addition, inherent problems in the PHC system that is being speedily introduced. PHC nurses are in the thick of things and ought to be allowed an independent role. They are central to defusing volatile situations arising at health delivery outlets in the townships. Yet they are bound by rules and regulations and exploited as cheap units of labour in the comprehensive services.

Why are nurses being denied opportunities (which the doctors have) of practising as specialist nurses? Are they responsible for the economic downfall of the country to have posts frozen and to become victim to the state's rationalisation policy? These are depressing prospects. Official attitudes need to evolve.

NTOMBIZODWA

I should dearly like to revive the culture of the nurse-patient relationship because it is so poor, if not non-existent these days. Today's nurses are systematically more advantaged than we were; yet they blunt their own case when they complain endlessly.

They have a lighter work-load considering that we did sluicing and domestic duties as well as nursing: things are being computerised more and more for them; the working hours are not quite as harsh as ours were, they have better education, greater scope for jobs, improved housing and better health due to nutritious food intake. If only they could harness the positive aspects of patient-first ethics no matter what.

I have gone so far as to say that should I be taken ill one day then I should prefer to be nursed by my own children rather than fall victim to the nursing resources in a hospital where situations arise without warning of nurses walking out of ICU, a place where patient-lives depend entirely on the manipulation of machines. For those nurses to go out toyi-toying, well it takes the breath away. Do they see their cause as significant above the lives of their patients? If so, this union attitude is fatal for the nursing profession.

CHLOË

I've had a glut of achievements, so much so that I easily forget the half of it (laughs gaily). As a student nurse I was chosen to demonstrate to the co-examiner how each procedure had to be executed. This was done before the practical exams, for her to be acquainted with the details, since she would be accompanying the examiner from Pretoria. I was identified as the best in the group.

A feature of my career thus far is that whenever something had to be innovated it would be discussed and sooner or later someone would say "Let us call Cloë in on this." That is for me a personal triumph.

When Margaret Miles came to start the nursing process at Livingstone (1978/9) I was totally immersed in fundraising for Health Year. We were darting around in a frenzy, in the coloured and black areas of P.E., with begging bowls to the fore. In the midst of this furious activity Miss Kimber made the shattering announcement that I was to be reigned in.

She had said, "Call Mrs Sioux back to the hospital, her ward will be a model for Mrs Miles." When told on a note of rising alarm that I was totally involved in the fundraising effort, she had snapped, "I don't care about that. Call her back; her's will be the first modern ward of this hospital." So with magnanimous forbearance I had to change course in mid-air.

Here at Dora Nginza there was at one time a problem with burns cases, who were nursed all over the show, becoming septic in the process. Dr Malherbe, an extraordinarily agreeable man, worried about this and one day asked me "What can be done to ensure better patient care?"

Well, with any given opportunity to be creative I allow myself to take wing, getting recklessly excited in the process. With an air of sweet reason I began to harangue: "Well Doctor, we can zone this area here and let's see, we can change the bathroom to be used as a unit; close that door so that the ambulance people stop making it a walk-through; we can have the children nursed here…." I found that there was enough space to kennel an elephant.

Dr Malherbe's face lit up like a Christmas tree. He rushed to Mrs Orlayne's office urging her, "Go to Sioux, find out her amazing idea for zoning off a Burns' Unit because she's got it together like an architectural blueprint, ye gods!" Since the establishment of the Burns' Unit our burns cases rank as amongst the best nursed in the region.

One more achievement deserves mention, if only for the tremendous input and emotional assistance of a wonderful team of people. When I first started on the educational side I was truly appalled at the sparse resources. Education without resources is like a house where the electricity has been cut. Resources shed light on the learning process.

I worried at this problem as a dog worries at a bare bone. I talked to friends, colleagues and associates. It became a bee in my bonnet until eventually, inadvertently, I discovered that I had gathered in a support group.

After a slow, bumpy process of intense discussion fraught with potholes, we were able to formalise the group into committee structure. It culminated in the formation of the "Friends of the Dora Nginza Society." With a lively sense of collective responsibility we pursued the central problem of lack of funds to upgrade the shortage of educational resources.

Unfortunately, "red tape" prevented us – as hospital personnel – from raising sponsorship. The problem was overcome by expanding membership to a secular community body. The objectives were broadened to include the social advancement of the patients after discharge. This enabled the committee to improve their surrounding environs, all within the principles of self-help and total well being.

Our agenda now enables us to function in the broadest social sphere. A happy sidekick is that a platform now exists for wider participation in the social change occurring during our country's transitional phase.

The *FRIENDS OF THE DORA NGINZA SOCIETY* has survived pressures large and small to the extent that we are now planning the re-burial of Dora Nginza's remains in the grounds of the hospital named after her. This will be done under the prodding thrust of the wonderful band of people serving on the committee. In my head I can hear the cheers coming up should this exquisite dream be brought to fruition.

Finally, tertiary education culminating in the BA CUR is an achievement of no mean feat, especially when your background for such serious pursuits is a large, bustling family like mine, with a hard-working job thrown in. Tertiary study was in fact a long, convoluted, uphill road to travel. There were formidable barriers to vault over.

In addition to the nursing degree and a specialist qualification in orthopaedics, I plunged into developmental stuff like the Dale Carnegie and lately I've nibbled at Honours but was deterred by financial restraints. There were now offspring standing in line for a piece of the family budget so "Mother" had to throw in the towel.

I think that all of today's problems in nursing revolve around the manpower shortage, of which the supply must be drastically improved. Invincible barriers exist between us and the regional authorities. Whatever motivations are written by us, in whatever eloquent style, it comes to nothing, like eggs smashed against a concrete wall.

It is no secret that the last time a study was done on staffing at this hospital, that the outcome was one that I could not accept. I found the norm, which *CPA* [Cape Provincial Administration] had laid down for staffing in the region, totally reprehensible and I am about to give up on the problem. I had made my views clear in writing that the norm ought not to be based on what is required for the small institutions dotting the regional landscape. The regional authority had replied that a situational analysis would be done. But all my effort came to naught at the end of the day - so much wasted effort on my part. We remain hideously understaffed. And I have no power to change that.

EUGENE

There's no particular achievement that I can claim credit for. Not even when in the 60's I went around the Cape Town hospitals collecting data required for the compilation of the proposed four-year course. I cannot claim credit for that because you see we worked as a team. Whatever you did individually, the credit went to the team so that the educational input collected was in fact to the credit of the Nico Malan College team.

There are many things that nurses do as part of their duty and no one bats an eyelid about it. Another thing is that the people at the top are forever emphasising that you are merely doing your duty. There's hardly guidance from top level, certainly no recognition, and praise is a foreign language that no one higher up seems to have heard of. Humility is a quality drummed into nurses as desirable, so they have come to accept their outstanding interventions as part of duty.

This has been happening all the decades of the century.

So much so that today, when nurses are required to write incidents to compete for merit bonuses or for promotion, they are hardly able to identify incidents because they were never encouraged in any way to blow their own trumpets. No one was ever called simply to hear the words, I like what you have done or well done! Quite apart form getting recognition, the everyday appreciation for things done well was never there.

I would like to see specialisation areas. The four-year course should cover merely the basics in all the disciplines. For the rest there should be scope for specialisation.

The other thing that I would like to see is the allowance of upward mobility in the area of specialisation. Part of nursing will always have to do with being at the bedside and there should be specialist nurses as there are specialist doctors at the bedside.

Then too, far too much irrelevant material is packed into post basic courses. It is simply too wide, as though nurses are not really sure what they want, as though they have some identity problem and therefore reach out to all the academic disciplines to try to have it all.

There are too many insecurities within the collective psyche of nurses. Every tiny little feud can pit one nurse against the other. Look what happens when tutors visit the wards. Instantly friction is sparked off like electricity off live wires, yet the tutor is a specialist in her field. There is too much hypocrisy amongst nurses, too much pomposity. We have to ask ourselves why we feel threatened so easily?

The status factor, which can be tormenting to subordinates, is largely to be blamed for many of the unpleasantries. And this is not only in the upper hierarchy. Amongst our selves too, nursing's aura of authority provides a kind of lever by which nurses find they can trample on those beneath them. When caught in a corner we hastily retreat behind rules, not always successfully I hasten to recall.

This is a frivolous incident but it illustrates the point I've just made.

Some years ago we sat in committee to decide on regulations for uniformity in dress. This was to become C.P.A. policy, which is still standing today.

As far as earrings are concerned, the decision was that only a pair of stud earrings would be permissible. And then one day along came a nurse with two stud earrings in one ear! The memory can still raise a blush in me, how easily a nurse was able to skate around *our* rules.

As far as uniformity of dress is concerned, it will be increasingly more difficult to stamp out individuality if that remains a desirable goal. The fashion ethic and the professional ethic have become so enmeshed that nurses find themselves in competition with bank tellers and office workers and in fact the culture shock is upon us as younger nurses display complete nonchalance to the "rules".

It is my honest opinion that the caring component is dwindling from the face of nursing. We're so stressed – the people in charge of wards – that we cannot stop to assist the little ones to learn the caring aspect.

The other thing is language. The patients come from diversified backgrounds and yet we are only bilingual, mostly English or Afrikaans, despite the fact the Blacks are in the majority by far. The fact that South African basic education did not pave the way for multi-lingual communication is truly bewildering.

Nursing education needs to re-evaluate culture as an educational need. How else can the nurse be adequately prepared to deal with people from a cultural milieu different from their own? Lack of caring and understanding in this regard has caught us in the deep.

I think a powerful thing is setting an example. We never know how many people we influence. It's a joke when someone says: don't do as I do, do as I say, but young nurses require good role models. It is an epic test of character that we provide such models in ourselves. Which brings me to a negative incident I'd like to share.

The people who were part of the committee that collected educational input for the 4D course, I know for a fact that there were people in the team who did not have matric, who were qualified tutors, because matric was not a criterion in those days. Yet they could achieve what they did despite their thin academic background.

With the proposed new four-year course they prescribed ridiculous subjects. The physics, maths and chemistry that they didn't have, they then demanded of the new nurses. I have a problem with this alter-ego type of existence.

The things I know of these colleagues I am talking about, is that when they undertook tertiary education starting with matric, which they had to scramble for in great haste, their subjects included Bible studies and criminology. Yet now they were imposing all this heavy science on the kids, setting a cracking standard they themselves could not have followed.

Somewhere along the line nurses suffer an identity problem. Someone will have to sit down one day and dip deeper into the essence of professionals. There is too much suspicion, confusion and uncertainty. Somehow I believe that we've lost our way there.

NOMPUCUKO

My special achievement was to innovate the putting up of drips by trained nurses. This happened after I had completed a course in mothercraft at the Glen Grey Hospital in King Williams Town. There were expected to put up drips on very sick babies, sometimes dirty babies from the rural areas with herbs compacted on their scalps. Sometimes these babies were moribund on admission and we had battle to put up the drips.

LAHLEKILE

When I returned to Frere Maternity I was keen to put up drips, as these babies were clean with veins clearly visible. It would be a walkover for me. However it was still regarded as a doctor's task so I had to make my request diplomatically. My colleagues were stormy-faced and berated me for plunging them into uncharted waters but I am immensely proud that professional nurses were allowed to perform this procedure because of my thrust.

I should like to change the outlook of administration especially as far as salaries and hours are concerned. The unsociable hours of nursing is an issue that can split families asunder. No one is keen to do nursing these days, certainly not my own children who suffered at not having their mother at home. One is forced to treat one's family with an attitude of neglect. We hear that change is coming but it is as slow as the formation of a stalactite.

LAST WORD TO LINDA

There is a disquieting slogan arising in the township here in Gugs (Guguletu – Cape Town) and elsewhere. It is *ONE-BULLET-ONE-NURSE,   ONE-BULLET-ONE-DOCTOR.* These are new rumblings here in 1993.

You ask me why? I can only surmise! I have an idea that it springs from a misperception about primary health care, which has not been adequately explained to the people.

Most of the information that people on the ground have is incorrect, subjective and dangerous. Besides, everyone is in a survival mode right now.

For instance, in the Day Hospitals, while you are busy with your dressings, someone will come in and take whatever he wants from the trolley because he has to participate in health care (bubbling laughter). He or she needs to be seen doing that and the service providers have no say. This is the misperception. Undeniably too, there is the lack of discipline in the entire atmosphere.

Take Gugs as an example. Here "the element" wants to rule the place. The nurses, with popping eyes, will say "While I am working with patients, like your own mothers, I am busy as a professional and I cannot allow you to tell me how to do my work, that is not how things are done."

This response could be perceived as belligerent. It could be an ominous signal to "the element" that nurses could be annihilated by violent means and we've all read in the papers how three or four nurses were burned to death in the 1992 strike (Transvaal area).

It seems to me that a segment of our youth is throttling itself with it strident militancy, its open contempt for traditional values. And who are in the first line of defence? : Mothers, wives, and girlfriends. What we need is a cultural revival. What we seem to be getting is a mass uprising. This could eventually have our noble profession on the ropes.

MID-CENTURY NURSES TAKE A STAND

In Chapter 2 the mid-century nurses (many of whom are still in practice) have told their story and during interviews did not shy away from discussing their position with candour, particularly those who have accepted early retirement.

They reject with equal contempt the contention that they were "Ja-baas" people. They have made an invaluable contribution, have suffered cruelties and injustices and, as borne out in their biographies, various individuals have challenged the system, either from within the existing statutory structures or on a one-on-one basis in the work situation. They remain undaunted. They are not going to allow the unfair criticism of today's nurses to eat away at their lives.

They feel that the analysis of the striking union nurses has not gone far enough into understanding the nursing situation of the oppressed people of earlier times. Nor do they seem able in this post-modern period to conceptualise the UBUNTU in which nurses' acquiescence was inextricably bound.

In moving on to summarise the experiences of these nurses it is hoped that their contribution to nursing will be marketed to a whole new dimension. As their parents before them had lifted them over the great divide, between tribal and modern life-styles, so to it will befall the forth generation of nurses to elevate the profession, out of the jaws of apartheid, into a new formation. South African nursing could then be transformed into a liberated, democratic profession, in step with universal professionalism for the 21st century.

Doreen Merle Foster

SUMMARY OF EXPERIENCES AND TRENDS

Anthropological

There was widespread belief in supernatural causes of ill health. The witchdoctors, or Sangomas, played a central role and were consulted before medical personnel.

Christianity was widely practised. In the Western Cape with its large Muslim component there was religious tolerance to a great extent.

Norms and values were instilled into children; firstly by grandparents, secondly by the siblings of the parents.

When a parental death occurred the family provided a support network, often on the maternal side.

The birth of a female meant joy to a male parent since the labola custom would enrich his economic status.

The drudgery of housework spoiled the growing, learning years for some, particularly in non-African cultures where families were bogged down by poverty.

African children were not allowed to come into contact with death and were sent away from a house where a corpse was left to "lie in state".

Marriages between people from different tribes were possible but not encouraged. For example, a Fingo marrying a Xhosa could be less favourable.

Social life in Cape Town was marred by the skolly element.

In rural and peri-urban areas of the country people resided side-by-side, learning one another's languages, until the Group Areas Act separated them.

On the whole children were not given a free choice. They had to rely on the decision-making of parents. In extreme cases a girl could have a marriage partner chosen for her.

Rural area people were largely of peasant stock living off subsistence economies while urban area people were mostly a working population scraping poor incomes off mining, textile and other industries.

Education

Teaching was an accessible and admired profession. Literacy was taken to the oppressed population through the contribution of teachers.

As far as the interviewees were concerned, the Good Hope and Cape Education systems were considered superior to Bantu Education by great leaps. Bantu Education caught some girls of the period on the cusp of their schooling years.

Corporal punishment was a factor.

The black child had to walk immense distances to school, often barefoot, without breakfast or lunch in some cases, depending on school feeding schemes once or twice a week for sustenance. In isolated areas some had to cross rivers and bridges to get to school.

Bantu Education imposed Afrikaans in a manner not acceptable to the people. Subjects like mathematics had to be taught in Afrikaans by teachers to whom the language was as foreign as to the pupils who were expected to learn by means of it.

LAHLEKILE

CHAPTER 3 - LATE CENTURY NURSING

PREAMBLE

The nurses of the late century period began their early schooling much along the same pathway as their predecessors. They walked long distances, often barefoot, mainly in groups and usually without the barest sustenance to pop into their mouths. Absenteeism affected the morale of the group. An exception was in the cape Peninsula and similar urban centres where community schools saved children from having to walk those endless distances.

These children were deeply affected by apartheid politics, which burst over their lives through the many legal acts such as the infamous Group Areas Act, a socio-political dagger that virtually obliterated their many cultures. One graphic example was the forced removals from District Six in Cape Town. This Act thoroughly eroded the cross-cultural community, which lived there in close cohesion. Children were not unaffected by the turbulence of state cruelty against their families.

They were a generation who at secondary level of schooling were confronted by further political turmoil. Countless numbers found themselves up against "Bantu" education, which imposed a kind of rote-learning system devoid of educational development. This brought so much racial hostilities and animosity that the tragic consequences resulted in "Soweto 1976". Those who could not accept "Bantu" education were flung into job-hunting which proved extremely debilitating both in industry and commerce where slave wages (for very hard work) sent a shudder of revulsion through the intelligent young people seeking their place in the sun.

In Cape Town, schools such as Trafalgar High, Livingstone and Harold Cressy, had grounded their learners in the socio-political perspective.

Consequently, children collided with a violent arm of state when they took to the streets to protest against the arbitrary removal of progressive school principals. These leaders were suddenly replaced when the notoriously unpopular "Coloured Affairs Department" came into being. The community dubbed the replacements "Stooges".

The appalling arrest of the children who were trampled, crushed and bundled into police vans and removed to Caledon Square raised the ire of the entire oppressed population of the Western Cape.

At secondary level there was little choice as far as academic subjects were concerned. Girls especially, were encouraged to do domestic science and needlework rather than maths and science, boys to do woodwork and gardening. Career choices were limited, mainly to teaching, nursing and policing.

Families tended to be large and poor. There was a raging hunger for education since doctors, lawyers and the like were erupting on the social scene as role models.

In the Eastern Cape Province, by way of example, a Dr Bokwe visited the historical Welsh High School while some interviewees were attending there. He made inspiring speeches to raise their awareness for the need to study further.

Unfortunately, tertiary education was an economic burden that most families could not undertake. Nursing then had an obvious advantage. However, the conditions of service and the exceedingly low salaries were piercing obstacles of such weight as to be almost unbearable.

Before the nurses of this period tell their life experiences the reader is invited to peruse the following overview (17:43-44) of the nursing struggle of this time.

1961:

A strike was organised by the hospital Workers' Union at King George TB Hospital in Durban to protest an incident of corporal punishment of nurses by a matron. Skilled and unskilled workers supported the demands that the matron be fired. They furthermore demanded equal eating facilities, proper food, the establishment of an employment insurance fund and an end to racial discrimination in the hospital services. Over 300 hospital workers participated in the two-week strike. As the police cordoned off the hospital the strikers were supported with food from the local community. The strike also received international support. Some of their demands were met, others ignored. Twenty-one of the strikers were fired.

1973:

Student midwives at McCord's Hospital went on strike for higher salaries. They were earning less than R40.00 a month.

1978:

The Nursing Bill published in 1977 was enacted in 1978. Although the Act makes provision for a non-racial nursing Council, only registered nurses who are "South African citizens" are represented. This excludes many black nurses who are, in terms of South African law, "citizens of independent homelands."

1979:

According to the 1979 "Race Relations survey" (as quoted) dissatisfaction among nurses over low salaries and poor working conditions was rife. In October it was reported that approximately 200 nurses employed at the Old and New Johannesburg General Hospitals resigned because of low salaries, late pay cheques and poor working conditions. The hospital authorities denied the report, but nurses interviewed the following day said the reported figure was correct.

1979/80:

Hospital worker organisations were formed in Natal, the Transvaal and the Cape. They aimed to break down barriers between health workers by bringing them together in one organisation. These organisations accept all hospital workers as members regardless of their skills and level of training."

LAHLEKILE

The nurses now proceed to relate their working biographies. It should be noted that though every attempt was made to interview nurses in the "Homelands" very few were accessible due to problems concerning strike action and general inaccessibility.

Where postal interviews were arranged, for example with nurses from kwaZulu Natal, registered mail was returned.

Telephone communication similarly proved to be most difficult. In editing the interviewee's stories, I submit the political axiom that, *An injury to one is an injury to all.*

Whatever happened in nursing during the apartheid era, affected all nurses in South Africa.

PART 1 - EARLY CHILDHOOD

CONTRIBUTORS TO THIS SECTION

1. Jane [a British nurse]
2. Nonceba
3. Pamela
4. Mynoena
5. Audrey
6. Billy
7. Rita
8. Joy.
9. Esme
10. Nomamobali
11. Magadelena
12. Euclid
13. Alfred
14. Peter
15. Farieda
16. Denise [now a Canadian]

JANE 1961

My name had no special meaning. To talk about my background I should have to go back quite a bit. I went to school in England in a small place called Hornchurch, which has the connotation of the spitfire pilots of World War II.

I started at the local school when I was four-and-a-half years old. In England they didn't mind what age you started as long as it was around five years. Then my father decided that for a better education he would send me to a convent school –the Ursine School – where I had to write a different exam because in England the education system was bisected into secondary modern for the not-so-bright kids and a grammar school for the more academic. I think they've stopped it now because it's a bad idea from the start, one sector believing that they're actually not as bright as the other.

So while everyone else from our vicinity went to the local school, I stood out like a sore thumb by going to a different school and writing a different exam. We were three kids in all, who had to walk down the village to catch a bus for a distance of about 20 miles, which at that time was an enormous stretch.

Our uniforms were different too from what the local kids wore. We were decked out in fancy red with a blouse and pleated skirt and a posh hat thrown in for good measure.

The secondary modern pupils walked down to school at the same time and we had to walk through them to reach the bus. Obviously we were regarded as the aliens infringing on their territory. This was one of the larger social features of my upbringing (said with a Colgate toothpaste smile).

NONCEBA

My name is Nonceba. My elder brother was seven years old when I came along as a "surprise". My father gave me a Xhosa name meaning "mercy" but later in my life I decided to give myself the name of Mercy in the absence of an English name.

I grew up with my maternal grandmother on a farm. In early childhood I had a great fear of cows and at school the teacher would use these bovine creatures to threaten us for misdemeanours. I was terrified. My fear spurred me on to work hard and it paid off with good results. From upper primary school I was able to learn in an urban environment.

PAMELA 1962

I came from a little village in the Transkei called Mount Ailiff and I had my early schooling there while for the rest I schooled in Umtata.

Those were pleasant days, I can't complain, though we had to walk to school because there simply was no transport of any sort. We walked three miles either way to school but there were others who had up to a five-mile stretch. We were almost all of us barefoot since our parents were not earning much in those days.

What I remember vividly from my school days was the dark cloud, which fell over us in 1949 when I was a little girl of about nine years of age. It happened that the principal announced one day that things have changed at the Post Office. He said only white people could use one door and "Non-White" people the other and that this would be the case everywhere in the country. He said, "So please children, do not enter the Post Office without looking up to see which door you – as a "Non-White" – will have to use.

Tiny as I was, that rankled. My mother had a small home industry and her sewing parcels swung back and forth from as far afield as Durban. I was the luckless child chosen to carry out the postal side of her business.

While previously everyone had stood in the same queue in the Umtata Post Office, suddenly there was a white and a black queue. Whites who arrived long after us were served immediately. The air would steam with our anger but when anyone ventured to protest, the Afrikaner lady would open the hatch and shout spitefully, "Wag julle beurt!" (Wait your turn!). I simply cannot forget the raw injustice of those days.

MYMOENA 1965

My name is Mymoena, shortened to Muna in intimate circles. I was born in the month of February in summer. In Muslim society our names are given in the social or historical context of the time and "Mymoena" means "the fortunate one."

I was born in District Six, grew up in Cape Town where, in the turbulent years of the 60's I entered high school. The 60's were extremely volatile years in our history. District Six had been a highly unique, stabilised community and I grew up there with children from diverse cultural backgrounds, some whose parents hailed from as far as Russia.

Going back to upper primary school days. I remember waking up to the dismal day when all the African children were gone. Their people had been the very first element to be extracted from the community and it felt as painful as though a prime molar had been uprooted without an anaesthetic. Then came the day when, with deep misgiving, we found that all the Jews were gone.

And soon enough so were the English and other Europeans. Their removal is a spiritual brutality, which remains vividly on my mind. Little did the Nats know that District Six would remain as a sore thumb amongst their iron fists.

To a child this forced removal was highly confusing. It was hard to cope with the intense feeling of abandonment when playmates suddenly were gone, whisked away by legislation. I remember sitting for exams in a high state of anxiety, having to travel by bus, having diarrhoea, and in fact failing hopelessly because of this enormous social change which had been thrust upon us so unceremoniously.

District Six was a unique place where everyone "belonged." Old people were looked after, children cared for. When the Nats destroyed this place, shunted everyone out to Mitchell's Plain 30 Kilometres away, it was described in the mass media as "The greatest piece of social engineering since Hitler."

Despite the removal, or the trauma of apartheid, my school years were wonderful. I began at an Anglican school – St Marks 0 in William's Street just up the road from home. The high school too was a stone's throw away, one of the historical schools of Cape Town, Trafalgar High.

In this outstanding school in the days of Mr Steenveldt, we were well grounded in a socio-political perspective. Besides, our own very cultural community was immensely supportive to the school.

LAHLEKILE

When the notorious "Coloured Affairs Department" came into being, the principal was forcibly removed. It was felt that he had been too influential in opening our eyes politically. They actually replaced him with a Coloured Affairs "stooge" causing the school to explode in uproar.

We students went out en masse picketing our protest in the streets, an action which was not tolerated by the state. All of us were bundled into police vans and taken to Caledon Square Police Station where we were pushed into jail, placards and all. Our parents had to come and get us out.

Fortunately most of the parents were open-minded because in their hey-day they had been drawn into struggle already, fighting for rights, so they understood our cause and gave us their solid support. In my own home my mother used to let us sit down after supper to discuss what was currently popping out of the newspapers and to put a meaning to it all.

When the time came for me to choose a career there was not much to choose from: nursing, teaching and domestic work seemed to be the only options. Perhaps because I am an Aquarian, I have a deep love for people so it was more natural that I should have chosen nursing.

AUDREY 1965

My name is Audrey Kanyisa. Kanyisa means, "to bring light." To my parents it was a matter of great pride and joy as I was their first baby. My father died when I was 9 years old so we had to go and live with our Granny to allow my mother to join the workforce.

From Granny's house the school was 7k's away. We walked the distance in groups, all of us barefoot. If one child was absent for any reason it affected the morale of the group because we relied upon one another for support throughout the journey-by-foot. We had no lunch to take to school, a further hardship relieved only on certain days when a feeding scheme provided sustenance.

Most unfortunately the next school we had to attend was even further away but we had little choice since the first school stopped at Standard IV.

At 12 years of age I was sent to live with relatives, not a happy solution. For the senior secondary years again I had to change horses in mid-stream, this time landing up with a new set of relatives.

It wasn't easy those years, money ever lacking. Then I went to do teacher training. When I left the training school I could not get a teaching post other than having to go to some remote spot, hardly a speck on the map and there I fell victim to the capricious system of a headman. Sometimes I was paid by courtesy of his lordship, sometimes not. This went on until 1959 when I thought, "enough is enough."

LAHLEKILE

BILLY 1971

I was named Belinda from the film "Johnny Belinda" and grew up under the nickname "Billy" which prevails to this day. We lived in the North End of East London and thoroughly enjoyed the rather notorious characters whom you had brought alive in your play of the same name. (Reference to the drama "North End" written and produced by the Editor of this work in 1991).

The golden school years are unforgettable, especially for the adventure of being escorted over St John's Road each day by the colourful traffic officer characters, Bill Goodford and Mr Carvalla. They were enormous men who took turns to herd us across. "Uncle Billy" would growl at us to make haste as he kept the cars at bay on our behalf. These days when I see Mr Carvalla quietly sitting in a corner at my geriatric clinic I have difficulty in reconciling his present image with that of the vibrant character he used to be.

RITA 1973

My name is Rita. I was born in the township of Alexandria but spent the growing years in the Transkei. There I was raised in church schools up to matric because in the Seventh Day Adventist Faith the children had to be imbued with our religion at the same time as being educated.

There were no taxies or other motor transport available to us so I had to walk long distances. Fortunately the world was still a safe place to be. There were no dangers such as child abuse or molestation by strangers.

JOY 1979

My name is Joy Nomvuyo. I grew up with my grandmother because of the early death of my mother. We had no contact with my Daddy in the early childhood years because he had settled in Port Elizabeth while we were in Peddie. We met up with him again when I was eleven years of age.

When we moved over to my father in 1965 it was difficult to get a place in school. My father was working and he had no wife to ease the burden for him when he had to accept the responsibility of two little daughters.

It was a deep and vexing problem for a man to have. I could never trivialise what my Daddy had done for us. With hindsight I see him as honest, charismatic, even far-sighted, for he made decisive interventions until we were able to take control of our own lives.

It was only after two years that I was finally accepted in school but made to repeat Standard II. Despite this setback I was amongst the top Standard VI pupils in the Eastern Cape, passing with distinction. For matric I progressed to the Newell High School.

Unfortunately I fell pregnant half way through matric, a tragic victim to the conflict between mind and passion. It was a wrenching experience but, because my father did not grill me relentlessly, I managed to complete matric after the baby's birth.

I then applied for nursing but found a huge stumbling block in the way. Baffled and bewildered I learned that weight was a factor considered in one's application.

LAHLEKILE

Though I had the striding gait of the long-legged, I was more than 70kgs and this was taken as excessive. My perishable body was standing between me and my dream career.

After three long years in the wilderness I was taken on and commenced training in 1979 at the Livingstone Hospital.

I was relieved of course since we had a financial problem in that my father was unable to attend to all my needs.

ESMÉ 1976

My early education and in fact up to Std V was in Afrikaans after which I attended Harold Cressy, one of the traditional historical schools of Cape Town. We were only Standard sixes at the time and I came first out of all the classes. I was clever those days (laughs) but the brains flopped a bit afterwards.

So my school life was good. For economic reasons and to help the family I wanted to leave school after Std VIII but my father engaged me in a very serious discussion. He said; "They can take everything away from you, but not your education."

To me my matric years were the best of my schooling. It was nice, I learned a lot and we had very good teachers, like Helen Keyes renowned for her skills as an English teacher. There were the train rides to and from Cape Town through the tunnel (mischievous smile on face). Oh, those were the good days!

NOMAMOBALI 1976

Actually my name is a Xhosa derivative but since that name is rather a tongue-twister for many, people have generally preferred to use my English name Sylvia, which I do not know the meaning of.

Nomamobali had significance for my mother. It means "stories." When my parents were courting my mother had a very difficult time. I understand that my father was a tomcat in his day, and was moving around a lot. He was born and bred in East London while she came all the way from Queenstown. One can imagine the difficulties that such distance apart must have caused the courtship.

Besides having many girlfriends in East London, my father was immensely popular within the family, so much so that the in-laws rejected a "foreigner" for him. This is how they saw my mother.

So when she got married there were marriage difficulties emanating from conflict with in-laws. It became worse when she produced only two sons, a fact which depressed her, as she desperately wanted a daughter to relate to and to whom she could confide all the stories of her courtship and marriage.

At one time she turned feral and bit an in-law on the nose. Another relative is running around with one breast, so much did my mother have to fight to get my father for herself.

That is how I landed the name "Nomamobali" so that one day I could be her confidante. Up to this present day whenever I myself am confronted by marital ups and downs, she always finds her way to me and comes to be supportive.

Early school days were spent in a rural area outside East London where we had to walk barefoot. The concept of a pair of shoes was a far-off dream. These school years made life as hard as winter because we had come from an urban to a rural environment, something so foreign to our lives up to then. Things improved vastly when I came to move to Johannesburg.

MAGDALENA 1977

Mine was simply a name, there is no particular history attached to it except that I was named after an aunt.

I was a good student all the way to matric and won some prizes along the way for academic achievement. During these school years I excelled in some sports, notably long jump, high jump and athletics. For the latter I gained Border and Eastern Province colours.

After matric I discovered that I would not be going to a university as I had planned. I had this colossal dream of becoming a marine biologist but this was not to be; the family budget could not take the strain. That was a grisly fact I had to face.

We were a considerably large family – twelve children in all – and I was one of the older ones. To complicate matters, those days we had slender options, unlike today when scholarships and bursaries are available.

My mother's dilemma was that in the event of them sending the first batch of children for tertiary education, we would have been five there at one time almost, something of an economic impossibility and she could not make fish of the one and fowl of the other.

As a point of interest, this is exactly what happened to the younger lot of the brood. All five of them are at universities today and it would have been six had my brother not already qualified. So I scouted the prospects and was unsettled to learn that one had to choose between teaching and nursing. I grabbed nursing in desperation; or rather it grabbed me because my mother arranged everything up to taking me to the station for the trip to Cape Town where I would commence training. To me the idea of nursing seemed as pleasant as castor oil to a healthy child. It was not really what I wanted to do. The train ushered me out in a daze.

EUCLID 1978

I was born at Frere Hospital where my mother had a fillip in being attended to by a beautiful Greek nurse whom she consulted about my name. The nurse suggested ***EUCLID*** after a Greek mathematician who rose to fame in the years BC. Well, I have an enormous sense of fun and of the absurd and I was comfortable with maths at school, so maybe a soupcon of dust from the revered ***EUCLID*** rubbed off on to me? (A thunderclap of laughter splits the air).

One of the reasons why I decided to do nursing was basically that in the socio-political situation where one's choice could fall on teaching, policing or nursing, the latter seemed the more attractive option. Given a choice, I would have become an entomologist, after speaking to an entrepreneur at Westbank who manufactured insecticides.

The whole plan fell through the mat when a white guy came along wanting that job. He took it up for a while but did not pursue the entomology studies, by which time I too had abandoned the idea.

ALFRED 1985

It's just a name. I'm from the Tswana culture. I do have other names but I prefer to use "Alfred", as the other names are not easy to pronounce.

I grew up in the rural area of Rustenburg (he smiles at my exclamation, Rustenburg being a "right-wing" area). It was okay in the villages (placatory tone of voice). I did my matric in Johannesburg then went on to university for my nursing degree.

PETER 1986

My father belonged to the apostolic faith and I was named Peter John after the Apostles who were the dominant favourites in his church.

Childhood was a dreadful time, an unspeakably dreadful time strewn with deprivation, unhappiness, parental bickering and hatred of each other. This was compounded by the death of my grandparents, later of my mother, and severe survival problems under a father who had not only become inflamed by alcohol but who slid into incoherent, bumbling, dysfunctional parenting.

I was 14 years old when my mother died and was forced to take charge of the brood – we were six in all – with the baby only two-and-a-half years old.

The family history, which preceded my birth, was pretty dismal really. It begins with a grandmother who, as a young girl, found herself pregnant from a white man. The discovery was inopportune, as the man had already returned to his country of origin somewhere in Europe.

In his youth my father was a soccer enthusiast. While travelling to every nook, cranny and dorp to play soccer he met up with my mother in Kokstad, which was predominantly an Afrikaans-speaking place. She too succumbed to puppy love and became pregnant. This time the social dictates of the day imposed an MGM (must-get-married) on them. They were an unlikely couple but they took the bull by the horns anyway.

Of course the marriage was fraught with pitfalls. It might have been easier to mate a lion with a crocodile. The conflict, which brewed from the start, soon escalated into terminal animosity. Their constant hissing and smouldering at one another created a hateful, brash environment, which was not conducive to child development and growth. Yet strangely, my mother's death emotionally kneecapped my father whose behaviour deteriorated almost from the moment she closed her eyes for the last time.

For the duration of an entire year I slogged at housekeeping, cooking, laundering, shopping, caring for the children while also attending school. The odds were colossal. I failed dismally. Then I decided to shut my eyes, harden my jaw and brought our plight to the attention of the Child Welfare.

We were given to my father's eldest brother but we didn't get much love and support from them. It became atrociously clear that they were in some financial difficulty and our welfare grants filled the deficit. It was no easy ride, but at least we had a roof over our heads. I became more restful, being able at last to look out at the world and began to make my way in it. For me to achieve at school – to come in the first three – something I managed from Std V right up to matric – was the most fantastic thing.

When I reached matric I decided that instead of going on I would leave school because the family were all leaning into me with wide open eyes and ears. We wanted a home of our own. My father was clearly petrified of taking the responsibility so I opted to be a Good Samaritan and left school.

Around March and April the realisation leaked into my brain that job-hunting was a staggering humiliation, which could go on forever without any success.

The last straw on the camel's back was when my baby sister came along to confess her rampant misfortune in having an unplanned pregnancy. I sat up as though on springs. The feeling was strong that the entire family ship would sink unless I did something to empower myself.

Propelled by economic insecurities I then went back to school and finished matric in a fragile state of mind. I had a spell at a Teacher-Training College, which I enjoyed tremendously but because of financial difficulties I decided that nursing was the only way. It offered an opportunity for me to be financially independent and also to become an independent person.

FARIEDA 1986

I was born in Stanger on the South-Natal coast. My first three years were spent in the care of my grandparents. When re-united with my parents we lived on a farm at Haven Hills from where we moved to Wentworth where I began my Schooling.

Today my parents are separated though not divorced. I met my husband at Wentworth and we got married five years ago. Recently my husband was transferred to East London and I'm quite happy to settle here in the Eastern Cape.

LAHLEKILE

PART 2 - LATE CENTURY NURSING

Contributors to this section:

1. Mr T
2. Hazel
3. Enid
4. Valerie
5. Irene
6. Ella
7. Esmé
8. Magadelene
9. Euclid
10. Flo
11. Rita
12. Joy
13. Alfred
14. Peter

MR T. 1962

My nursing career began rather late, preceded by teacher training at the Heald Town College in Fort Beaufort. Unfortunately those years were hard as winter due to the "Defiance Campaign". All of us were opposed to the Nationalist Government with its system of Apartheid

At college we were deeply affected due to frequent police raids on the premises. They often came during our meal times, a busload of them. From the moment of their arrival we would freeze into a tableau of apprehension. They simply invaded the place, shouting threats from the stage, pouncing on certain individuals at any time. Their character was not conducive to peace. It only served to strengthen our resistance.

During these years there was a law that forbade blacks to walk in groups of more than five. This was a law which I experienced first-hand. We were robust adolescents in a tiny rural town and it was natural that every opportunity would be taken to paint the little town red.

One Wednesday afternoon a group of us were walking along the streets as merry as crickets. We were munching fish; quite a luxury for fish was only available in Fort Beaufort on Wednesdays. It was great fun strolling the quiet streets, boisterous with horseplay. Until we were accosted.

The thugs in uniform that evoked reprehensible law, hurled us into the van like a sack of potatoes. From there we were shoved through the door of the police station while their power-mad eyes invited student provocation. We remained there crouching in corners until the Heald Town authorities came to intervene by which time we were running sore, feeling wounded, incapacitated.

Teacher training during 1953 - 1956 was disturbing because suddenly a sentence-method, akin to rote learning, was introduced. We were expected to pioneer this as an introduction to "Bantu" education. We were the unfortunate targets chosen by government to slip the sugarcoated capsule of inferior education to the black child.

Naturally we recoiled from the idea. That was a turbulent time in our history. We students could not stand aloof - some of us became recklessly excited. Daily the tension built up. I could feel it, coiled within me like a spring moving to breaking point.

LAHLEKILE

Well, when a fox is trapped he gnaws off his leg to be free. My peers and I took Bantu education as poison to the black child. We were not prepared to commit a moral crime against our own people and so the majority of us left.

The phase of job-hunting was very depressing. After a series of short-term disasters I became thoroughly street-wise. At a butter-and-cheese factory I was referred to spitefully as "the learned Black" and at a department store I earned slave wages without any economic incentives.

My parents were unable to do anything for me during this dismal time of drifting but they were uncritical, believing that I would surely climb high up the social ladder. They believed in me. When the door to psychiatric training opened I tried my luck and was accepted for training in 1962.

We did not have tutors and were taught by professional nurses. There was no method. They read textbooks to us and failed to make psychiatry interesting to their students. Fortunately the psychiatrists delivered the main lectures. They would give us assignments to do at home then expect us to relate what we had learned to our peers.

My teaching ability soon became apparent. They pounced on my expertise and I had to explain things to the class. They believed that when one shares relevant information with others, in a learning situation, that one then gains fresh insight into the process of sharing. From then on my interest in psychiatry was fired.

HAZEL 1967

My place of birth is Uitenhage but the wonderful years of senior schooling occurred at Trafalgar High in Cape Town. Since those days at "Trafs" the name "Hazel" fits me well because of my proficiency in sport. Everyone knew the name as a result of athletic achievements for the school.

Unfortunately I missed the heart-thumping excitement of today's youth for we were not given access to the range of options currently available for sport-talented people. I do not have Western Cape or provincial colours, trophies nor any memento except the name, which to my peers, means great renown for outstanding athletic ability at school.

I commenced nurse training in 1967 at Groote Schuur Hospital. It was a career choice influenced by my mother who provided interesting information and anecdotes concerning nursing. Somehow her information steered me in this direction though truthfully I lacked motivation. Again one has to note that things have changed, in that children are these days fully informed by means of attractive enticements such as "Open Day" activities for the various professions.

The training itself was progressive. It made me pleased that I had come into the nursing profession for it provided space for further growth and development. However there were countless difficulties sprouting directly from the question of race and colour. The matrons were power-figures, wholly prejudiced, and politically warped as far as I'm concerned. Their dislike for the so-called coloured nurses was overt. They placed themselves on such remote pedestals as to be unreachable to young girls like ourselves, who had to grapple not only with horrific situations of patients in the stress of disease, but with all the personal uncertainties of young adolescents cast adrift in this specific world of adulthood.

There was an absolute lack of matron-nurse relationship; similarly a lack of senior nurse support for their juniors. I had a senior nurse who taught me how to lie out a corpse, which happened to have been the body of a male of massive proportions. To me, a teenager fresh from school who had never even seen a naked male, the shock was tremendous. The experience goes down as the most awful, the most indelible of all the negative experiences during training. In fact I broke down. Yet there was not a single person in the nursing world at the time that could help me still the torrent of tears. In the final analysis a doctor showed compassion and came to calm me down.

I believe that the overt racism influenced my training negatively and quite needlessly. We were terribly abused as "coloured" nurses. To illustrate this contention I remember how they used us on night duty. It suited administration to use coloured nurses to nurse difficult cases such as the cardiac sufferers. One time I took a stand here. Quite boldly I stated that if I am not good enough to be seen nursing white patients then I shall not do it under the screen of night duty. A matron told me in a voice that was metallic that we were on a par with maids.

We were deprived of opportunities to study further. That was a major injustice. After all we were young, perspicacious and intelligent. Even if you had the courage to ask, you were pushed out as though you were a hound out of the rain asking to be allowed into the lounge.

Meanwhile white nurses were encouraged to go further. Whites – most especially Afrikaners whose bloated egos were fed by the system – became sisters-in-charge and sister-tutors while the administration did its collective darnedest to keep us down.
Fresh from graduation they could rise rapidly while most of us were kept for years and years as "staff nurses."

This is precisely how white "superiority" became institutionalised in South African nursing. The apartheid paradigm dominated nurse thinking. Turning this around is not only a matter of practical urgency but of justice.

The overall difficulty was that we were not allowed to speak up for our rights. One of the matrons – a Miss Squire – was particularly infamous amongst a cadre of professional tyrants. She bullied us mercilessly over misdemeanours with uniform.

Now one of my personal idiosyncrasies happened to be a taste for fashionable, distinctive clothes. I liked to indulge myself wearing attractive garments and actually poured money into the acquisition of a good wardrobe. The nursing uniform seemed to rob us of our very sexuality. Moreover the caps were simply repulsive. In fact, one's self-esteem could easily disintegrate with one glance in a full-length mirror.

My training occurred during the "Twiggy" era, the time of the mini-skirt. Now a student nurse would not in her normal senses wear her uniform to the radical length that the fashion of the time dictated. I have not encountered a single incident when anyone went to such lengths…pardon the pun. What we wanted, one and all, was to have the next best thing, a length a fraction above the knee.

Miss Squire – a human prune whose odd proclivities we had to cope with – appeared to derive great personal satisfaction in stopping nurses at every public point. She would yank our caps and make it bigger and we were expected to walk around like Victorian fossils with helicopters on our heads. It was an abuse of our personal dignity.

ENID 1967

I was called Enid because it was a traditional name (she gathers her shoulders into a delicate shrug, eyes dancing merrily) and any other might have passed my parents' imagination. I was one of six children and it is possible that they had simply run out of names.

School years in the small town of Graaf Reinet were pleasant at primary level but at secondary level the realisation sank in that we were not getting the best of the world and that bred frustration. We were not getting the education that our counterparts in the white schools were getting (she allowed her voice to trail away on a note of distaste).

I went into nursing because of poverty. My father died after a long illness with gastric ulcers. My mother went out to work for the Boers (pronounced Boors) from dawn to dusk. The seven of us had to come from school and fend for ourselves. It was impossible to educate all of us beyond secondary level. That's why I went into nursing, but even then it was not easy for us, we didn't exactly get it handed to us on a platter.

I commenced training in 1967 at the Conradie Hospital, in Cape Town. My training was very strict under white tutors, the principal an Afrikaner who subsequently left to run a farm, so you can just imagine. She ruled with a rod of iron.

At first we were accommodated at the Conradie Hospital then it was decided that because it was a white area we could not be kept there in the Nurses' Home. Transport was then provided to shunt us backwards and forwards between Somerset Nurses' Home where we were made to reside and the Conradie Hospital where we trained. Nobody seemed to regard this arrangement as abnormal and that is how it remained until I qualified three years later.

I remember an English-speaking tutor as well. She used to say one thing and mean another and she was hypercritical too, very conscious of her "supcriority" as a white person. Instead of nurturing her students she threw us to the wolves.

VALERIE 1969

There were such few Indian nurses, no more than a drop in the ocean. We wanted to be part of the spectrum. I started at the newly built R.K. Khan Hospital in Natal in 1969. There were no African trainees, only so-called Indian and Coloured. As all the units were not yet functioning we went to the King Edward by hospital bus for part of our clinical experience. We lived in the R.K. Khan Nurses' Home.

At the King Edward we were totally integrated as Blacks – 90% Zulu – speaking girls, 10% Indian and Coloured. It was my first experience of racial integration, a huge culture shock, for I had never encountered the Zulu culture in my life, having come from the Eastern Cape.

We learned serendipitously to respect other cultures. This was not required by the *Searlian ethics we were taught. Nothing about other cultures in our land could be found in any of the books. We learned at the bedside and by talking to peers. We learned that we could not serve fish or eggs to the patients in the lying-in wards

* Reference to Charlotte Searle, a South African Professor of Nursing as this was contrary to Zulu custom. Similarly we were not allowed – by tacit rule – to remove the traditional strings around the abdomen and right wrist (some kind of skin was used to make these strings).

I learned how important the elders were and the profound respect extended to grandparents, among the first to be shown the newborn. It was the same with Moslems. The Imam had to come and whisper messages in the baby's ear. It was taboo to allow people into the nursery, a "no-go" area at that time. Yet we had to bend the rules, to gown and mask the Imam to let him in.

This total lack of a holistic approach in nursing education is lamentable. Nothing is more important than for nurses to have the various cultural practices opened up so that these limitations are avoided.

IRENE 1971

When I actually looked up the meaning of my name I learned that it means "peace". My Mom used to call me her "lucky charm" and that was a good omen that worked for me. We didn't all have rich parents; our household had nine children in all so it was not possible for the parents to take us all beyond secondary level. I was the fifth child, and also the lucky one chosen to go as far as matric.

Being her "lucky charm" my Mom chose me to run important errands for her whenever she needed special assistance from an aunt or other relative. She believed in me and I rarely let her down. Whenever she caught me up in a fond embrace thoroughly pleased that my mission had been successful, she would cry, "My lucky charm." I then felt as snug as a puppy in a deep dream.

My school years became difficult the higher I went. In Standard VI we had no choice in getting academic subjects. I disliked needlework but shivered in joy over mathematics. The teachers of my time were excellent. At one time I discussed career prospects with the history master. He steered me in the direction of social work to which I was amenable, pointing out with grotesque logic that nursing was a "dirty job."

The main factor that drew me to nursing was the financial advantage in earning money while being a student. That could only ease the burden at home. Besides that, I really loved people having always had a caring attitude, so I took to nursing like a duck to water.

LAHLEKILE

I commenced training at the Conradie Hospital in 1971 but we blocked at the Nico Malan with the Groote Schuur nurses. We had a problem with this in that the Groote Schuur nurses had an attitude about training at a superior hospital like "Grottes" and they always made out that that somehow bestowed superior status on them. Conradie was a small community hospital in comparison.

But the dice fell in my favour because I was a top student from the beginning right through to the finals. We had lovely tutors, Judy Moses, who was so proud to have us being the first all-matriculant group. She was a Somerset trainee, very motherly to us. Our class teacher was Charlotte Maponga, whose brusque sense of humour had us skipping through anatomy on waves of laughter.

So we had very good years as nursing students. The Conradie girls were like one big family. We were always referred to as "Die plaaskinders" (the farm children). Our seniors were very protective towards us.

The only fly in the ointment was an attitude emanating from the auxiliary nurses who gave us hell, saying we thought we were the bees knees in nursing, but a lot of that stemmed from personal unhappiness because they had had the opportunity to train, yet had not been able to get through the finals.

ELLA

In 1959 a calamitous disaster struck our family when we lost my father in a fatal mountaineering accident. He was 39 years old at the time. Mummy then had to go out to work when I was seven years old. So through the loss of my father the caring side of nursing appealed to me.

Later on I met a lady who greatly influenced my decision to enter nursing. In fact it was you. (Editor). I used to look forward to hearing you tell interesting stories about people, your encounters, and your friendships. You had such great collegial relationships and I wanted those things for myself.

I did my training at Frere Hospital in East London. Actually there wasn't a choice because of family economics. I felt very supported both by the ward staff and the college. They nurtured me.

It was at a time when the hospital was still extremely autocratic. Matrons and sisters were giving young nurses an exceedingly hard time in 1971. A new order was winking from the wings but the hierarchy was still very autocratic and in fact, vestiges of the old attitudes have survived to this day. It was never quite shaken off, we can still quote the American adage: "If you're white you're right, if you're brown get down; if you're black get back." (Author anon). Today in the nineties, *we* still have to stand back.

There are two sister-tutors whom I remember well, Mrs. Mbalu and Mrs Mtyeko. Mrs Mbalu is remembered for her favourite word, "normally". What a dignified lady. Both were simply great teachers.

LAHLEKILE

ESMÉ 1976

Teaching was definitely not for me because of the slight speech impediment in which I am unable to pronounce the letter R clearly, and still cannot do so.

During training they made me feel <u>that</u> small (hand gesture indicating a slender space between thumb and forefinger). In fact on the first day they made me stand holding up a drip for about an hour. The sister in the ward that I came from did not telephone the sister of the ward I was sent to, to say that they were sending a patient along so I was made to wait until they could ride out their ire.

They were excessively strict those days, but also non-caring as far as the student nurse was concerned. Wherever and whenever they could put you down they would do it. That's our so-called Coloured nurses at the time when I trained at Grottes (Groote Schuur) in 1976.

You had your ups and your downs. I think many times my sense of humour helped me through. I remember the time when a matron came and spotted dirt on the floor and her reaction was to kick over the bucket. She did this with theatrical impact. Instead of getting all hot and bothered about it, I simply laughed. That was a survival strategy, to laugh my way through the snaps and snarls.

But there were times when your spirits plummeted after they had a bite at you. There was nothing outstanding either positive or negative that I can say about my training because things were well balanced. There was much more team spirit, like if you work in Casualty everybody would work the entire shift and then flop down together somewhere outside at 5 o'clock to watch the sun come up. So you had the bad times but there were fun times too.

MAGDALENE 1977

I started training in 1977 at Groote Schuur Hospital where the Barnard brothers were practicing at the time, Chris and Marius, the famous heart surgeons.

I did well theoretically, though the feeling was strong that nursing was not the profession of choice for me. All through training I vowed that as soon as my family were out of dire financial straits I would carry on with my life, doing something that appealed to me. It was a plan I willed upon myself almost daily.

After a few years I completed General but instead of spreading my wings I got caught up in the sorrows of a tangle of children clawing their way through basic education and a weary mother straining to make ends meet. What could I do other than nail my colour to the mast? And so after General, I landed up at Frere Hospital near home.

When I was at Grottes (Groote Schuur) there were no black nurses, meaning Africans. There were none at all, only Whites and Coloureds. The resentments in the depths among blacks and browns are beyond white comprehension, yet here is a graphic example of the conditions that sprout these unhealthy feelings.

The Whites had their college right next to the hospital while ours was in Athlone at the Nico Malan. So we were 100% segregated, furthermore by buffer zones, highways, factories, and townships. They used apartheid as a screen to hide from their eyes the vast reality of Blacks. Could we ever forget?

The nursing education was okay. You met an awful lot of people. There was a glut of matrons too, most of them Afrikaners who, from their cosy warp of white perceptions, gave us a hell of a hard time. She suddenly breaks into mirthless laughter. I remember an incident concerning this frizzy hair of mine. (The editor observes that her hair is honey-coloured, attractive in its frizz-curl and worn long, down to the shoulders).

I'm sure you know what the Cape Town mist does to this kind of hair? (More laughter, raucous this time): Those days frizzy hair was *out*. The Cape Town girls sported long shiny manes, which in the Moslem society resembled silk curtains hanging down their backs. Well, these "boertjie" matrons, reaching the heights of tactlessness, ordered me to stop walking around with frizzy hair. I was to straighten my thatch! I can still see their lips distorted by disgust. That was their attitude, which was not nice at all.

EUCLID 1978

I was the first male to do the integrated course at Frere and I was the second – after Ralph Sylvester – to do "midde" at Frere, the fifth in South Africa, hence my ANACCOUCHER certificate is 05.

I remember my midwifery training occurred when Prince Charles and Di got married. (The now late Princess Diana). I used to curse those moments when I was working in the labour ward and everyone was running to watch the wedding on T.V. Hell, you couldn't leave labour ward to go and watch T.V., no way. After that I worked in a general ward. This was after I was given an inter-departmental transfer. Eventually I landed in Casualty where I worked for several years.

Training had its good moments and bad, the bad mostly from the old dragons in charge of hospital administration; people who were the gatekeepers of the profession, people who could decide who would go forward in nursing and who would not. Their devastating power lay in their pens with which they could ruin young peoples' careers at the drop of a hat.

I had some nasty brushes with nurse educators in the college too because that was the time that they started to integrate Blacks and Whites. The educational facilities at Frere were traditionally divided, Blacks on the West side and Whites on the East side. Integration began when I was on my second Block. We were moved into a classroom where there were few English-speaking Whites. This was to boost the numbers, for the majority of Whites were Afrikaners.

Together with the sprinkling of Whites we then became a class of twenty English-speaking students. I developed a friendship with a white student who happened to be female and to the surprise and embarrassment of all, this perfectly human form of behaviour sparked a contretemps.

One of the college dragon ladies corralled me and asked whether my hormones were working in the opposite direction? I can still picture her shaking her head at the unfathomable behaviour of black people. "What do you mean?" I asked, truly appalled. And she began a semi-playful tirade with, "You're a bad influence on the girls." By means of facetious rhetoric it was conveyed to me that classroom mixing of races could not be taken to inordinate lengths. The textbook was the focal point around which social intercourse revolved and the buck stopped there. She wriggled out of the moral question of whether one was expected to be invulnerable to human friendship.

I then realised that I had had my wings clipped and that I'd have to watch *their* parameters from then on. They may have had great difficulty in conveying a clear message but there was no doubt in my mind that they had double vision.

They saw a numerical solution in getting a balance in the two official language groups while at the same time they were hell-bent on keeping the same groups socially and politically apart. This point was underscored by a vociferous nurse educator who had me on the carpet. She claimed that Blacks were having a negative influence on Whites through academic inferiority, yet the facts spoke otherwise for we actually got better grades than them more often than not.

To me the whole thing was a piece of rank triviality but you must remember that that was the time when mixed marriages and sex across the colour line was absolutely illegal and so friendship too, was remorselessly disapproved of. The unspoken code of conduct for the Frere classroom was: '*textbook mixing only.*' One wonders whether the dragon ladies will ever come to look back on these times introspectively?

Well, I did not believe in a non-existent challenge and so to everyone's immense relief I allowed the friendship to fizzle out. There was no emotional hemorrhage. I just saw the Whites as shortsighted and insular and found their racial paranoia inappropriate. Moreover, their analysis of human behaviour did not open up any paths for constructive change.

FLO 1979

I started my general training as someone who was a rather sweet, innocent, overweight eighteen-year-old. Full of trust and a firm belief that the world is a friendly place and that money grows on trees.

Well, sense was soon knocked into my mind, as soon as I wore my first pair of pinching navy-blue lace-ups, starched white uniform (too long) and white cardboard cap. Not to mention the hairpins, hastily borrowed from a suffering comrade.
The mirror seemed pleased. Now I was a "nurse" and there on my shoulders were proudly displayed a pair of mustard coloured epaulettes to prove it. What a profound shock lay in store for me.

The fact that no one prepares the novice for the shocks in store is actually quite worrisome from a professional point of view. From the start one ought to be warned that nurses operate within enormous buildings where the essence of life is played out as part of their daily routine – birth, death and every misery in between.

I was eighteen years old then. Issues like death and dying were beyond my coping skills. There was no psychological preparation for the impact of a dying human being on the souls of girls and boys fresh from school, no hand around your shoulders when the burden of life becomes too heavy; no ointment offered for the blisters on your feet; no support offered when you've been puking in the sluice room with the smell of your own vomit up your nostrils.

You've entered the adult world and thou shalt act accordingly. How fast you grow up when you've got to relieve another person from their excreta; when you witness a child being born; when you've got to tell a bereaved family a relative has died. On rare occasions you go home at night with a song in your heart when someone had smiled brightly or expressed gratitude for something. You then know that you've made some difference in somebody's suffering.

RITA 1973

I developed an admiration for nurses after encountering them during visiting hours at the Baragwanath Hospital. The place was like a beehive. I stood mesmerised in this action-packed setting, simply gaping at the nurses instead of focussing on the patient I had come to see.

Those days when you fixed a drip you had to stand on a chair to count the actual drops. I was charmed and envious seeing the attractive young ladies with complexions of every hue – pink, yellow, creamy-chocolate- so very beautiful in red-and-white uniforms which set them a world apart from us lesser mortals. No one was idling anywhere; they were happily buzzing about their business. That's what motivated me.

Of course I applied at once and went through a wonderful training experience at *Bara. The S.A.N.C. examiners had a rather tolerant attitude. For instance with catheterisation – they believed that you were doing the procedures all along and they were not going to fail a nurse merely because stage-fright made her clumsy. If you could handle the catheter in such a way so as not to injure a patient they would pass you ignoring the frills attached to performing the procedure.

Nurses from other hospitals who came to do the practical exams at Bara told us how they could fail at their home hospitals up to four times on a basic procedure such as bed-washing, simply because whoever examined them had a fetish about procedures being performed to their particular brand of perfection. Those nurses worried themselves sick over practicals and ran around like headless chickens.

* Barangwanath Hospital

At any rate their examiners certainly missed the point. With practical exams it is a matter of panic in a tense environment that could cause students to fail. Now that nursing claims to have modernised it self, examiners ought to create a calm, cogent, well-calibrated environment. It is within their power to break out of the stereotypical mode of examining procedures, this for the 21st century.

The training at Baragwanath was brilliantly absorbing. I most admired Mrs Nkhwanazi, the nursing educator who impressed me as having pedigree. She had a quirk about not being called "sister". Correct categorisation was of immense importance to her. She used to say. "I'm not "sister" I'm Mrs Nkhwanazi. Do you see a belt around my waist? Secondly, sisters do not go through the VIVA." She was referring to an exceedingly tough oral exam, which separates the academics from the ordinary sister-tutors.

JOY 1979

I loved nursing, most especially the interaction with patients. I enjoyed seeing them progress from disease to healthy states and mourned when they passed on. There was a 3-year general diploma course and a 3½-year course encompassing midwifery. I took the latter.

Training was quite absorbing but very difficult because of the amount of theory rooted in practicality. Within the first two months there was a mountain of assignments and tests, very exhausting and demanding, whereas we had been spoon-fed in school. So that was the first difficulty that I had to overcome.

Secondly, when coming out of block I was assigned to theatre. That was probably the worst part of my training. It was such a busy arena that orientation could barely take place. For a first-year student to be baptised in the waters of theatre can be only a cruel trick of fate. The strain is often more than one can bear.

I remember on the first day being in a place where the packs are autoclaved. The importance of this task lies not in its immediate consequent use but in the event of its making. We worked in an atmosphere of hushed disapproval.

There was a sister-in-charge – OOH – from the very look of her you shook with fear. She sent me to the instrument room to fetch a tray but I floated off, not knowing where the room was or how the tray looked. I just found myself standing in the theatre passage.

She eventually came looking for me and, knitting her brows in irritable perplexity she screamed, "Didn't I tell you..." There was a snap in her words, which I interpreted as a warning. I maintained a nonplussed silence, standing shivering in fright at the way she talked. The only question that occurred to my deadened perceptions was that I had to leave nursing. In the end I got used to the rough of theatre and stayed for two months.

Another difficulty was the telephone, something entirely foreign to my way of life. It rang unexpectedly and I picked it up, not knowing how to handle this thing while every nerve in my body was informing me that something had to be done. A soft "hello" from my throat eventually unlocked my paralysis.

The person on the other side leaped at me with a: "Have you never spoken on the telephone before? Nurse who are you? Come to my office at once." My heart was beating too fast for comfort. "Where is your office?" I asked almost pleadingly. "First Floor" was the terse reply.

That matron displayed an almost unheard of alacrity in chastising me while I stood sullen under her diatribe. I cried so much afterwards that I landed up in Casualty in a state of flustered dishevelment with severe epistaxes (nose bleeding). The incident had me enveloped in a blight of depression. I felt emptied of everything as though the shock of her scolding had atrophied all of my power to think, to feel, to rejoice.

ALFRED 1985

Training was interesting, lots of theory and practice but there was overload on the practical side and it was not structured. If you had to do 40 hours in a surgical ward for instance, it did not matter what you did within the prescribed time; whereas it ought to be prescribed that the student should do this and that and that. The emphasis from the legal point of SANC is merely on the time frame. That corals you. Even after writing exams you might have to go back to do hours laid down by SANC.

There were a lot of stereotypes. The initial problem lies with the attitude of people. There are those who underwent the apprentice type of training, spending three years in different nursing situations and they are confident in the practical work, one can grant them that. Somehow these are the people who seemed to feel dislocated by our presence, keeping themselves much at a distance from us.

From our side we were still students; we had to get information from them, have our work-books signed but the negative factor was that from our side, some people had that attitude that we are "degree" people and so, superior to the diploma nurses.

From both sides then a conflict attitude was sparked off. There was a hot bubble of confusion. It was expected that certain behaviours would be displayed – that one, because of an inferiority complex will behave a one way while this one, because of pomposity at being an academic student might behave that way. This could lead to confrontation even if one did not necessarily have complexes. Nursing ought to allow one room to be your self without all that needless pain of assertion.

During my second year at university the 4-year course was introduced. Now how it worked was that the college was providing the theory for the 4-year students and the university was preparing us for the degree but we were all doing practicals at the same hospital.

When the 4-year people came, from their side they had the satisfaction of getting more recognised certification in psychiatry, community, midwifery and so on, over a short period of time. That seemed to give them a firm psychological superiority over us, they believed. I think that if that were true, that it would be a bad prognosis for human progress. After all, we were struggling to improve our range of options by means of higher education. Yet they seemed baffled, surreptitiously besieged by us.

The older trainees on the other hand were wrinkling their noses saying, "These people are getting over 4 years what we did in almost 6. There is bound to be a reduction in standards." There was no objectivity, only this harangue that could demolish the morale of students in favour of the credo that served the collective.

Thus nursing rides three waves. Those who had more experience or wider horizons due to more courses were able to come down on us who had the academic vision.

And all students got caught up in the momentum of nursing without any thrill. Action for action's sake; over-scrupulously wrapped in rules.

What affected the learning process was that students were regarded as part of the labour-force. That is not right considering that the range of tasks carried out is enormous. If it is required that dressings be done, the students would suddenly be taught in pedagogical tones and then become their reliever on the line. And if they have enough people to give injections then they would not teach you the procedure because you are not needed for that. This assumption on which ward policy is based is insulting and naive.

The students are used as a workforce, so their in-service training is more related to the needs of the ward than the learning needs of students. I think this is disadvantageous for students. If students are to be rescued from having to cope unsupported with the complexities of health care delivery and the pressure of an academic course, then a new strategy is required, a quantum leap in nurse education thinking.

At the same time you cannot divide learning up into different compartments when learning is a process. You cannot say, "Let me learn how to set a trolley" because setting up a trolley will differ according to the situational dynamics. Having modules – the linchpin in training – causes the students to be driven like robots, performing tasks.

There was no specific motivation for nursing in my case. One was exposed to a minimum of 10 options in vocational guidance and within such limitation had to grab the option which most appealed. I wanted a helping profession and weighed the pros and cons. I was under-capitalised, halfway so to speak, and nursing had financial advantages.

PETER 1986

I started training in January 1986 at Frere Hospital. The train journey from my home in Durban to East London was scary. The journey took three days and I was a lone passenger going into the unknown. But when I got there it wasn't so bad. I was able to make friends speedily, being somewhat of an extrovert.

The first year was uneventful but the second was so filled with emotional turmoil that most of it was spent either close to tears or with a pounding heart. All because I met and fell in love with Tammy (name changed).

She was the sister-in-charge of a ward where I was assigned as student nurse. Our partnership evoked disapproval, which lay heavy in the air. Despite this we later got married and somehow she gave me a sense of security, of stability, something I needed as a result of my childhood experiences.

I then applied my mind to my studies. Okay, I never got distinctions or prizes during the four years of nursing education but that wasn't of prime importance to me. The major priority was to get through.

The principal at the College was my mentor. She did not know this but I admired her so very much and wanted to be like her. I also had two other tutors from my own community who took me through most of my subjects. To the students they were in fact the driving force propelling our growth. It was most enjoyable being in their charge. The class was "multi-racial" and this was the first time in my life that I met up with whites on an academic and social level. It was a tremendous adjustment for me because throughout my life I had not had contact with them at all and it was strange but nice too because the penny soon dropped that we are pretty much the same. A few of the students had similar backgrounds to ours and on the whole there was no discernible difference.

I had previously had the impression that whites were superior because that's what they wanted to be. My attitude was cool, if that's the way things are then fine, let them be superior. But being in one class with them I soon learned that they had no claims to superiority on grounds of skin colour. Being white was simply a horribly strong advantage for them. We had white tutors too but they were a different kettle of fish. They overtly concentrated their energies on developing their own race group, asking questions of the white students while blotting us out of existence through indifference.

Naturally there were problems inherent in the situation. I was determinedly ambitious and felt that to make myself heard I needed to behave proactively. We were six blacks in a group of 36 and we always huddled together until I devised the strategy to split us up in pairs and spread ourselves more evenly through the class.

My peer colleagues supported me in this move but it was to no avail. We remained invisible to the white tutors. Their attitude made me feel emotionally disadvantaged but through personal determination to succeed I forged ahead, becoming rather pushy in class, because I was so desperate to learn. I had a total conviction that I knew where I was going, that I wanted to develop my talents and potential.

EDITOR'S NOTE

In appearance Peter is white, having descended from a European grandfather. To a stranger it would be impossible to differentiate between him and any other member of the white race. His classroom experience underscores the deep rift between people in South Africa purely on grounds of race.

PETER CONTINUES

An enormous fly in the ointment was the nurse educators' response to my courtship of Tammy who was a staff member of senior professional status while I was a mere student. In fact it caused an unholy uproar. One of them approached me and ordered that it had to end.

This struck me as abominable. I had come to care for someone very deeply. How and why was I to end a most meaningful relationship? Their attitude filled me with such appalling anguish, which I was forced to bottle up and carry around with me. With hindsight I can see that they were overstepping their bounds.

There were no enjoyable experiences at College. I merely went through the motions, never taking part in concerts and cake sales that they had, not participating in sports day ...... I had already developed a steady relationship with Tammy and she was the most important thing that had happened to me, so nothing else mattered.

PART 3 - THE PRACTICE YEARS

MR. T (1962)

Remembering my promise to my parents I wended my way upwards through many different courses, also a nursing science degree, plucking too the ripe plum of Honours, in psychiatry

As for difficulties, there is a sack-full. My actual interest was in the clinical field whereas I was placed in administration. There are so many changes in current practice that the administrator is little more than a go-between, unable to develop subordinate staff. Colleagues pulling from behind you are often resistant to change. They got scared taking risks.

The greatest fear is for a mishap to occur which could lose them their job or maybe put them in jail. Now is that helping a patient? You need to accompany the handicapped person as caregiver, giving assistance and support on the road to recovery. It is lethal to keep a patient dependent on you. When you interview the mentally ill it must be as partners, neither one dominating the other. In this way you bring understanding to the patient so that despite the handicap, the person can discover self-reliant skills that can help him or her to become functional in a normal society.

The difficulty is to get supervisors and caregivers to adapt to this viewpoint. In supervisors there lurks the perpetual anxiety that a "master" will be calling and are you managing your department? Some people are too concerned with the hygiene of the patient or the cleanliness of the ward. You see nurses squawk and scramble like hens to please the supervisor who may exclaim; "Oh, I see the patients are sitting on the step" or "I'm so pleased that the dormitories are fresh and clean. It causes me a quiver of grief that this tradition had not perished a hundred years ago.

The domination of people with tunnel vision is another low in nursing. There was a time when reading a newspaper to a patient was an offence for which you could be expelled. Nowadays it is believed to be therapeutic.

By far the greatest difficulty concerns resistance to development. Service providers often balk at having to upgrade their knowledge and skills. They're satisfied to give instructions and to do things for patients. There are very few who cherish the ideal of quality care. This is very sad. Colleagues do not want to be shaken out of their comfortable ruts so that their minds can unfold its marvels. As a result of this attitude, institutionalised hypersensitivity abounds.

This aversion to progress applies to other departments too, such as those who supply goods to nursing services, like Sores. The people there display apathy so that it could take you five years to achieve your goals in work.

For instance, you could requisition a change in beds. The motivation is that a steel bed is unsatisfactory. Let us have a wooden bed with an inner spring mattress just like at home. The dangers of a steel bed are pointed out in writing.

When this order goes through to Sores they say, "Oh they now want to turn this place into a hotel." This kind of drivel is an irritating response to a serious innovation from administration. I found that the bad attitudes of low-level supply workers are an incredible obstacle to the speedy recovery of the mentally ill.

MERCY 1962

Well, my training at Livingstone was enormously interesting. I went into it with my eyes wide open. What struck me quite forcibly then was that nursing is strongly dominated by a religious compulsion in the form of Christianity.

The standard of training was high. Remarkably, there was not a single black tutor and the senior matron posts were held by whites. The only posts held by blacks were the sisters' posts, equivalent to today's senior professional nurses. Those days they wore veils. That was the highest position held by a sister. When I was about to do my finals the first black tutor came along, a Miss Sauli from Grahamstown.

We had a tutor called Miss Slater who subjected us to little cruelties all the time. Her face resembled a sour lemon most times. There was never a smile for a nurse. If you were doing your best as an excellent nurse then she would find a way to have you at the short end. Woe-betide you if you were poor, for then she'd make your life miserable. Always we worked in a climate of tension and obduracy.

Her favourite accusation against Blacks was that we share our beds with bugs. In tones of freezing rebuke she would shout: "Come and do your work properly! All you know is to share your bed with bugs! When I first heard that it sent shock all the way to the soles of my feet.

So we had a terrible life because of this person. At any rate we did well. Whenever results came out it was published interdepartmentally. It was an occasion for our juniors to jump around like toads in a thunderstorm. They'd come and peruse the results critically, hoping to put down loudly anyone who failed to do well, throwing their comments all over the place. Of course this spurred us on to excel both in theory and practical. Anyone who plonked a practical could not very well laud it over juniors after that so we applied elbow grease to our studies.

JANE 1961

I always wanted to enter the medical field. At five I wanted to be a brain surgeon, at six a doctor and in fact throughout school I had a burning ambition to become a doctor. My father turned his axe on this idea, expostulating about the "long, long training" and what was the use when in the end I'd get married anyway?

His arguments were strident enough for me to decide to become a physiotherapist instead. For this you had to do orthopaedic nursing first. You were accommodated at Birmingham for two years and could then apply for a bursary to train as a physiotherapist after which you'd work for a city municipality for a specified time.

In the event I liked orthopaedic nursing so much that I backed off from physiotherapy and readjusted my goal. I commenced training at 17 years having started school early and having left after 0-levels, which is the equivalent to your Junior Certificate. I had no desire to go to university. That was in 1961.

I loved nursing from the first day. There was one tutor whose influence was paramount. She taught us anatomy and physiology, which was quite involved in the orthopaedic hospital. She was prim and proper, staid and dry. I cannot remember her name anymore but certainly her face. She approached me once, saying, "Haven't you thought of doing medicine? Because your marks are good enough." However positive this made me feel my brain became sandbagged with studying after a bit.

Those day's things were very strict. You went on the ward and you kept your mouth shut. My most vivid memory of those days concerns my sojourn in a surgical ward. Remember the old wards that took the form of a big annexure, a veranda? – The old orthopaedic ward at Frere is similar to that.

The sister's desk was smack in the middle. There was a duty room but the sisters preferred to sit in the centre of the ward with the sluice room on one side the dressing room on the other and they carried a glint in their collective eye.

So you worked in an atmosphere of tension and gloom from the minute you hit duty till the time you went home. You had to be busy or at the very least look busy, never sitting down. We were persona non-gratis.

I vividly remember on one side of the ward were drips. There they hung, all along the whole side of it and it was your task as student nurse to watch all the time that they didn't run through.

In those days we counted drops at the speed they were running at. If it happened that they ran through – which they did with the old bottles – they would actually run quite a long way down the tube before they stopped short and this was an appalling nursing crime. It drove sisters to the utmost fury.

If you were a registered person you'd simply get a syringe and sterile water and then just push it up again before putting your vacolitre in. If you were a student nurse, first of all new, you'd get a tremendous telling-off and then Sister would say, "Right you, tap it up." And you'd take your scissors and wind the tube around it with your fingers and it would take you hours to tap it up. It was a big sin and you couldn't get away with it. They were so strict it was suffocating.

Whenever there was nothing else to do we'd go and clean bedpans, scour floors or shine lockers. There were people who did the house-cleaning chores but we were encouraged to do anything and everything. There was no camaraderie, such as I see here amongst sisters and students. We were still under the military model then.

From 1967 to 1968 I went to work for a nursing agency in Chicago in a paediatric ward. When I returned to England you still had a military model in the early 70's, but interspersed were people with a fresh attitude, who were beginning to loosen up.

At that time one could note changes in the uniform too. When I started training we had the whole tootie – a dress, which had an apron on top and a bib, which you had to pin so that the pin did not show through. We were expected to wear these with the grace of a Roman toga.

The belt was something else. Student nurses wore plain, starched belts but in England upon registration, we had elaborate belts with a particularly ornate buckle. The buckle was something precious that your parents, husband or boyfriend would get for you. There were a large variety of patterned buckles to choose from. This ornate buckle represented an ultimate dream, no longer to be scolded or disciplined in any way. It was your very special thing. It's hard to guess if this tradition is upheld anymore.

In addition we had cuffs. When you came on duty you rolled your sleeves up and put on these cuffs. The collars were detachable and that had to go on as well. Then there were different caps for each of the three years of training.

The caps started off with huge pieces of starched material, which we had to fold, turn around, fluff out and then perch them on. Of course if they were too small or too large you got sent back to redo them. That was very much the military model. We lived in fear and trembling. The intention was for us to become independent, responsible and tremendously efficient.

MYMOENA 1965

Numerous difficulties arose in nursing right from the start. One could not get to the matrons, the untouchable guards at the gates of nursing. Should you have had a pressing problem it made no difference, they were so unfriendly, so unapproachable. In a caring profession that ought not to have been.

The colleagues, doctors and patients were a source of happiness, since I love people very much, but the institution itself stank. It was like a factory, utterly impersonal, devastatingly so for the young student nurse.

The food that they provided defies credibility. What were we given at teatime after starting so early in the morning and working so hard? A slice of golden syrup bread; in our own homes we did not have such meagre fare.

And then for lunch we were not allowed the facilities in the dining room, which were strictly for white nurses. In my third year a change occurred when the facilities were opened up but along apartheid lines. What then masqueraded as lunch? Nothing other than boiled eggs with a slight variation on Tuesdays when a watery curry gravy was poured over the eggs – yuggh – "egg curry" it was then called.

Each day the thought struck home: How was one to continue enduring this purgatory? I consoled myself: "Never mind Muna, when you finish your training the sun will come up and you shan't have to take this any longer. Well beyond the 70's this deplorable menu remained in vogue at Grottes. The apartheid dining room practice came to a sluggish end only now, in the 90's but it will remain a blot on the history of Groote Schuur as long as we all shall live.

As a Muslim nurse it was doubly difficult for me because during Ramadan, time and again I had to break my fast. The great distance one had to travel from home to work brought the hungry gremlins growling in the stomach. In winter it was tough. The problem was exacerbated by the means one had to employ to break the fast at a time when duty and prayer time coincided.

My solution was to take some things from home and at prayer time to sneak into the kitchen just to have a drink and something to nibble in preparation for the solid meal I would have at home hours later. Should a matron have caught me in the kitchen even with my own food, I would have got a verbal lashing for such audacity or may even have been dismissed. It is a cause for celebration that we survived the excesses of their dispassionate style of management.

I experienced a crisis or two, or more, while on district in the 70's in the Heideveld area where the people and the students were being shot. They lay in the streets beached like dead fish in an oil slick. It was my first experience of the multifarious brutality that infects our society as far as physical violence is concerned.

We had to hastily establish "safe houses" through an outside organisation I belonged to. We were then able to nurse the victims of the shooting under cover otherwise they could forcibly have been taken away.

The discord acted on us as yeast on dough. In the super-charged air around our heads we swung into action, transporting patients from the scene of the shooting to places in Claremont, Rondebosch and even the large mansions of Constantia where they could be nursed into recovery or re-evaluated for removal to other points.

LAHLEKILE

That was the 1976 revolt when we experienced the painful realities of life and death in an unprocessed form.

A similar horrifying situation arose in the 80's. A period of extraordinary volatility when again the catastrophes came thick and fast and we had to organise safe houses.

Our homes were raided but despite wrenching, agonising despair, we carried on, scrambling around to scrape together an arsenal of bandages and improvised equipment. We had to organise things in St George's Cathedral where we had to nurse the students, ever in the front lines; man the telephones, get food.

Every available public hall was opened up to get people safely in off the streets. Everything else became meaningless outside the momentous effect of the state's poisonous contempt for the people in-struggle. To me it was so incomprehensible it could well have been happening on an alien planet.

Hunting for food was very hard work. You would start at your own home, scavenging every cupboard, then go on to neighbours, relatives and friends. It would have been unlikely for us to sit down to warm meals knowing that a stone's throw away people – like at Crossroads – were unable in the circumstances to provide for themselves.

No, I was never "honoured" with promotion although I secured a post as senior professional nurse in later years. I was known to be an outspoken person, recognised as an offshoot of Trafalgar High and suspected to be an activist. I regard my lack of upward mobility as a form of punishment for believing dissonantly in the human right of freedom of speech for every person. I refused to "lie down" as it were. Of course upward mobility will be far easier for the young nurses of today.

PAMELA

One difficulty I experienced occurred after I passed my midwifery. I could not get a post at Frere Hospital and we had set up home in East London.

At that stage they were giving preference to black nurses above Coloureds. I could not understand the situation. What I learned afterwards, and I don't know how true it was, was that the local Coloured girls were "always falling pregnant, " with the result that they preferred the black nurses. My husband actually had an argument at work on the moral aspects of the issue, that the matron of the day, Miss Gleaves, had this power, to discriminate against nurses on a basis of skin colour.

The other difficulty was the astronomical difference in salaries between the racial groups. I had landed a post under the Local Authority and the difference between the white nurses' salaries and ours was so glaring that it made it difficult for us to cope with the demands of living. I mean everyone desires a good standard of living but we could not keep up with ours because of the huge deficit in salaries.

I remember at one stage I had a (uniform) frock, which had got too short for me. You know how it is when you get older, you feel that you can't wear the minis any longer. I couldn't really afford another uniform. So I let the hem out, only to find that the dress now appeared in iridescent dark blue and light. The old part of the dress had been bleached in the sun, and the new part had retained the original colour dyed into the cloth.

On the morning that I wore this particular frock I was damp with apprehension that people were going to hassle me at work because of the two colours. I thought of telling them that I was growing (delightful laughter) …and sure enough when I got to the clinic the alteration made a terrific impact. Incredulous looks were passed. I had to endure their contagious laughter and teasing and, with what dignity I could summon, I gave the rehearsed response: "I'm growing!"

There was a white nurse who was very fond of me, Sister Grim. She noticed that I had lengthened my uniform and when I seemed disconsolate, came over to chat with me. In the prevailing atmosphere I clung to her like a drowning man to a lifeboat.

When I let out the embarrassing tale of how I could not afford a new uniform on my extremely low salary, she listened almost unbelievably.

In fact she was quite stricken when she realised how much more she was earning than I was even though we were doing the same work. Moreover, she was a practising Christian so this incident affected her deeply. She felt – and said so to those in charge – that it was wholly wrong that there should be any difference in salaries on the basis of race.

Though the campaign for *a living wage* was constantly simmering on the political hob, I'd like to think that she may have had a little to do with the change of heart that the authorities underwent in the course of time. I should like to believe too, that they could not have realised what the low salaries were doing to us, the relentless erosion of hope and confidence that is the legacy of poverty.

There was a time when I suffered tremendous discontent over the issue. This was while I was working in the TB service. You become discontented when you ask for an increase in salary to enable you to keep your head above water, and are given a cold response – sorry, we cannot oblige. If you can't accept this then you will have to vacate your post – well I couldn't give up even the pittance that I was earning and had to manfully swallow defeat. I left the service later but for other reasons.

MR T

One night while on night duty in the clinic I had an emergency call. It came from the centre ward. The hospital had different divisions for separate categories of patients, the physically frail separate from the psychotic and so on.

On this particular night I found staff and patients milling around a wide open door, which had me worrying that patients could abscond. A suicidal patient was standing in a pool of blood. It looked like a bowl of rhubarb pudding had capsized on to the floor. The patient was extremely violent so the nurses had left the door open.

Everyone stood rigid. The entire room was humming with tension. Once he saw me his towering rage began to subside. "I am going to die," he said, with a note of finality. It was astounding to witness a life ending ludicrously, formlessly, dribbling away into nothingness. I said to him, "What can I do?" I spoke in a manner that would allow my words to soothe him as warm water adding, "If you are going to listen to me then I shall help you."

For a few seconds he chewed that, swallowed, and made a gesture of complete helplessness. I extended my hand. Infinitely slowly he began to respond, allowing me to apply digital pressure, then to carefully stumble him out to the clinic, saying with deadly seriousness, "If you lose more blood then you're going to die. We are trying to save you from dying. The doctor is coming soon but first I shall have to clean you up and apply a bandage.

He let my words hang in the air. Then his lips contorted and he said, "Please ask the others to go away." I got them to do so, leaving only the two of us and the nurse who had alerted me to the crisis. When the doctor came he examined the wrist and began the arduous task of stitching. The patient was then bedded for the night, transferred to a general hospital in the morning and returned later that afternoon.

The following day he asked that I be called. The moment he saw me he spoke out in a voice marvellously clear "If it were not for you I'd be dead now" he said. That moved me deeply. He was a tall, hefty man who scared everyone with his toughness but it was just by the spoken word and a rope of trust that our minds had been able to make a deep – cutting communication.

I shall refrain from mentioning some of the crises which I've experienced since it could be flung back in the teeth of service providers. Moreover I am sensitive to the violations of the dignity of life. Let us leave the skeletons of this type of nursing in the psychiatric cupboard and instead work for change.

BILLY 1971

One of the difficulties I experienced were the meals given to us at Groote Schuur, unlike at the Nico Malan College where we were well-fed, with three-course lunches and hot coffee at bed-time, enhanced by fresh koeksisters sold to us by one of the housekeepers.

At Grottes we had to stay in for lunch when on straight shifts. I think that there they were under the impression that they were feeding birds. A Sunday meal could consist of a slice of bread, a piece of lettuce and tomato. I used to think mournfully, "Gee, at home my mother would be having a sizzling roast on the table, not to mention chicken pie or hot curry and here am I with *this* on my plate?

At Somerset where I did midwifery the food was nothing short of a disgrace. We'd nibble a few mouthfuls out of necessity and scrape the rest into the pig bins, so the pigs were well fed. What passed for meat no one could be sure of. Some say it was kelp. Nurses like putting names to everything so we called the thin sliced meat "platvleis" (flat meat). Seven-singles was the name applied to cut and fried polony while the Somerset meat, which resembled marine flotsam, was termed "seaweed."

Another difficulty was racism. My first job was in private nursing but I came smack up against the apartheid, which was so rife at the time. All the cases that the white sisters did not want were foisted off on us but I wanted jobs around town as they were getting. The Alexandria job (near Port Elizabeth) was on a farm where at night one could stand outside and see the lights of Algoa Bay but I felt far from inspired and uplifted, knowing that I was being pushed around where others were loath to go.

When I applied to Frere and was accepted for theatre nursing I discovered that the apartheid there was simply appalling. We had to work in the ground-floor theatre set aside for blacks, whom they referred to as "Non-Es." The fifth-floor theatre was reserved for whites to the point that we were forced to go there to request instruments used for delicate eye or ear ops. The staff would be as nasty as could be, saying things like, "Oh what do *they* want it for?" Yet they'd handle the costly, fragile instruments with complete nonchalance unlike ourselves who would package it most carefully on roller towels so that the points were protected.

Whenever new machines were brought in, it had to be dispatched to the white theatre with the old ones then passed on to us. When inevitably the time came for us to work in the sacred white domain the very first thing we were oriented to was "the invisible white line" in the passage. We have to work on one side of that invisible line and white nurses on the other. We could cross if we had to but always at the risk of being racially insulted. Dusting was done from the middle to your racial side. There were two defibrillator machines and you had succinct instructions on that, to use only the "black" machine on the black side.

If a doctor disliked your face life could be pretty grim. There were two so-called surgeons during my time at

Frere, who did a lot of damage in theatre, one a gynaecologist, the other an Irish surgeon. At one time the air conditioning was faulty so all the caesarean patients had to come over from the Maternity side; similarly the Gynae patients for hysterectomies. These doctors, apart from being thoroughly abhorrent racists, were incompetent too, working only on blacks, many of whom died on the operating table.

The Irish doctor had a marked brand of malevolence. There would be nothing wrong with what the black sister did but he would fling every single instrument on the floor in sudden fury. He could swear in a deep profane fearful atmosphere he conjured up, freezing us as though at the point of a gun. He stopped short of making a demented lunge at her.

There was no support from the sister-in-charge who merely spawned a homegrown philosophy that a surgeon needs to be given a sister whom he likes so that he can perform at his best. I somehow found it hard to go along with this belief, for the doctor then appears as cunning as a fox getting his own way.

The difficulties caused by race were endless for us. When the Cecelia Makiwane hospital opened I was in the midst of a theatre technique course. The problem that arose then was that we suddenly lost out on the big cases, which we required to complete our registers, so now we had to approach the white theatre to request permission to scrub there.

One day by arrangement I went to scrub for a major case only to find a white nurse, all gowned and scrubbed. She placated me by saying that the theatre matron had instructed that I be allowed to take over when the patient was asleep. Thoroughly peaked, I took my grievance to the theatre matron but she rapped at me, "Oh Gregory, you know how to set up a table, everything is basic, so you take over when the patient is asleep."

I found this syrupy patronisation wholly unacceptable and replied, "No thank you. Even if I know the whole procedure I still want to do everything for myself." She looked at me with a grim expression. I knew that I was marking myself as a renegade, yet I wondered why so many other students were prepared to put up with that kind of racial insult? She said, "Well you are a trouble-maker. And you're being difficult because that's the way things are done, you ought to be able to see what we are at."

It was worse in the orthopaedic theatre where one was treated like a leper. They had comfortable change-room facilities while we had to make do with the small closet used by working men as a resting-base since they had nowhere else to go. They would socialise there during their breaks with all our clothes hanging around. For morning tea the sister-in-charge would blow her self out like a peacock and call "Mrs P, go and make the NON-E. Sister's tea." It was hurtful to have to accept tea on a dull little instrument tray with crockery set on an acceptor bag and with milk that could have been yesterday's stock.

Doing the theatre technique course was again devoid of joy for us because of apartheid. We were four whites and four blacks. The funny thing was that none of us could ever score higher marks than the whites. We were ignored during lectures even when our hands were raised to answer questions. The lecturing doctors underrated us terribly as well. My anger made me see them as a soft set of parasites that fancied their white skins entitled them to patronise the world. I don't mean to be offensive but really, our values are different.

Then something happened which caused us to suspect that the test results were rigged. That is because only one black sister got 98%, yet all the whites got more. This is just an example of how sick racism can be. Anyway we passed theatre technique alongside the whites and in spite of them.

There were several crises as these are bound to occur from time to time in the operating theatre, almost as though it were an occupational hazard. A horrifying accident occurred when I was assisting the scrub sister one day. The patient was a young woman of thirty years who had come in for an ear operation. No omen warned us of the dreadful tragic event to come.

We had just introduced a new anaesthetic machine where the oxygen button instead of being on the right side, was now on the left. The anaesthetist was experienced at this job but I believe that when one works with smooth expertise it happens that you do not consciously think out every move. It's like driving a car or playing the piano – your hands work at their own volition.

The procedure for survival was to give a tiny spurt of carbon dioxide first, then to allow oxygen to run through, all under control of course, but on that day the patient did not commence breathing. I had already undone my gown so I looked at the machine in alarm when the patient failed to breathe. A cold shiver ran down my shoulder blades the moment I realised what was happening. On a note of panic I said to the scrub sister, "It's nitrous oxide not oxygen coming form this side." She naturally informed the anaesthetist at once.

He was appalled and sprang into frenzied action to reverse what had been done. The seconds were like eternity. I had to pass the drugs being used in the emergency, writing up meticulously what went from my hand to his. The muscles of my hand felt as though they had turned into red-hot wires. The patient was transferred to ICU where she died.

There was a stressful court case with a sour after-taste for the anaesthetist who resigned after the case to take up employment elsewhere. He had suffered a burning humiliation when the surgeon had failed to back him up, that it was a freak accident because of the new machine.

In the meantime I felt distinctly out of sync for being praised in the circumstances. They found that I had done outstanding record keeping under the tragic emergency circumstance. A residual thought constantly nags – was there anything I could have done to have saved her life? That crushing thought continues to percolate in my brain long after the event.

I experienced a corny happening during student-training days. I had accompanied a friend to the amphitheatre at Groote Schuur with a patient who was to be a model at a doctor's lecture. No sooner was the patient comfortably seated than a medical student approached us with a friendly grin. "Would you girls like to see the Receiving

Room?" he asked. There was nothing in his manner to indicate mischievous intent.

Like lambs being led to the slaughter we obediently followed in his footsteps, after all he was our peer, quite a handsome guy, moreover a medical student, so wholly acceptable in a social manner of speaking.

To our shock and horror he led us into a room where cadavers were lying on slabs, each with a formalin drip-feeding into it. He explained – cool as a cucumber – that formalin is flushed through to preserve and deodorise the bodies so that it does not give off a rancid smell during the dissecting procedure.

With gritted teeth and churning stomachs we followed him still, like treasure-hunters in an eerie tomb. He showed us a side table where brandy was kept. They were allowed one or two tots, obviously to boost their morale if not their un-solid stomachs for the gruesome task in hand.

Then we approached what looked like an enormous chest. It took up the length of the entire back wall. By that time I was so full of terror that I thought my skin would crack with it. We dared not look at each other, each one fighting to conceal her fear. As we got nearer to the chest my skin prickled and my hair stood on end. I could feel drops of perspiration on my bottom lip.

The moment came when we were forced to look and my heart stopped beating as my senses swam. We were looking at the amputated parts of the cadavers as it had been sawn off or cut out. Some of it resembled biltong, a delicacy, which somehow I cannot bring myself to eat ever again. The moment was one of petrifaction.

Our sick companion – for that he surely was – tried to draw us out in small talk but I felt the contents of my stomach coming up, nudged my friend so that together we high-tailed it back to the amphitheatre, letting our rasping breath return to calm before we re-entered the room.

Dr De Villiers gave a riveting lecture on Bells' Palsy, which I thoroughly enjoyed, soon forgetting the grim scene from which we had fled moments before. The amphi-theatre was refreshingly normal after our gruesome experience, with a lovely-liberated kind of atmosphere. We were able to giggle again, a delicious, infectious mode of behaviour. It was so enjoyable for us as nurses to share a learning experience with the medical students.

HAZEL

An extreme emergency happened one night when I was working in the obstetric unit at the Peninsula Hospital as the senior nurse-in-charge. This lady had come in at about the 36th week of pregnancy. Though the membranes had ruptured there was no sign of labour. We immediately instituted the monitoring, which included that of the foetal heart of course.

At one time, after she had been to the toilet, she came out running and indicated with hand gestures that something was happening in the birth area.

I got her on, to the bed and upon a cursory examination saw the baby's head outside the vagina. With great urgency I alerted the medical team and to my astonishment she was taken to the labour ward. Now this puzzled me greatly. Our most recent monitoring had indicated a strong foetal heartbeat and I was extremely perplexed as to why they were not taking her to theatre.

My anxiety level rose with each passing second as I waited for news of the patient. An hour later when I could bear the suspense no more I phoned Labour Ward and discovered with horror that they had in fact completed delivery but as an SB (Still Birth).

Mortified, I felt that this had been sheer negligence because that baby had been alive when the patient had left our care. Why did they not induce the labour? Why waste precious time attempting every which way to do the impossible?

In the end they had been forced to do a cleidotomy to make the delivery possible. Far worse, had I not run up to the labour ward on wings, the mother would have witnessed the sight of her headless baby lying in a river of blood. It had been an instinctive gesture on my part to shield her from this sight by very speedily covering everything up.

ENID

I had acute difficulties in my nursing career at times. I worked at Groote Schuur Hospital. At one stage there was an announcement by the government that there would be a pay increase. We were naturally excited. But then came the news that the increases would be only for our white counterparts. This news hit us like a thunderbolt. It was absolutely unacceptable, nepotism in the extreme.

As a result of this gross violation of our needs, our very humanity, we decided to stage a protest. I was one of the leaders of this protest in the early 70's.

We planned a sit-in on the premises of Groote Schuur. Our mission was to mobilise the intelligence and determination of the nurses, to get them to realise their capacity to be as outraged as we were, and to take action. Of course we had contacted the media so that our protest could reach the uncaring hearts of the highest authorities.

This did not go down well with our censorious superiors who immediately set about discovering who the "ring-leaders" were. They reported us to the SANC. As a result of that I was unable to find a job both locally and nationally. My service had been suspended and then terminated. Fortunately I was in the process of registering with the British Nursing Council.

I then put Cape Town behind me and secured a job in Johannesburg at the Jewish Home for mentally handicapped children; I got the job there only because it was in the private sector. All doors in the public sector had been shut in my face after the brief sit-in protest at Groote Schuur (her brows furrow as though in bewilderment). Following an application to the Coronationville hospital I had received a smack in the face with the following reply: "We have no vacancy for people like you in our establishment." I regard that as an act of malice.

So I worked in the Selwyn Segal Home in Sandringham while my papers were being processed for England. These I snatched up in relief the moment they were ready. No sooner had I settled in England when I was informed by my own coterie of friends and colleagues that my name had been struck off the SANC register. I was sent newspaper clippings verifying this appalling vendetta against me (at this point she failed to keep the astonishment out of her voice).

Fortunately their bigotry did not affect me at all. I happily carried on in a healthy, normal society, free of the iron-fisted rule of the South African nursing authorities. When I left this country I had about £30 in my pocket. That was what I had at Heathrow airport, with no one to come and meet me since I knew not a single soul in England. I wouldn't dream of doing anything like that now, but I did it then (her eyes glitter and she cannot keep the triumph out of her voice).

At one time I left England for a while to work in a copper mint industry in Zambia. My rationale was that I could then return home from that point in Africa. However my timing was wrong for the political pot was hotting up during a brief visit home in the ebb - tide of the apartheid era.

It was a time for me to reflect profoundly on the future. I found that I had grown so militant that I could not keep quiet. I would be unendurably unhappy under the status quo of nursing with its seemingly insurmountable polarisation between white and black. In the broader society, through the media, I came to realise that the ugly hand of repression was yet being raised.

LAHLEKILE

The year that I stayed in Zambia was an eye-opener as far as nursing is concerned. I found myself in a situation where there were many clinics strewn around with two hospitals for back up. In the hospital situation we nurses were left to diagnose and prescribe far beyond the scope of nursing according to "Western" norms.

When I got back to England I was in charge of a ward where there was a diabetic patient in the sideward. Her sister came to visit one day and reported to me with a quick frown of anxiety that her sister was "very sleepy" and was not responding at all.

I went in, saw all the signs and symptoms of a diabetic coma and without a second's hesitation I went straight for the IV infusion apparatus and set it up. It did not occur to me then that I was not on Zambian soil any longer. Only afterwards did the penny drop, when the nursing officer in charge said, "Do you realise what you've done? We are grateful that you saved her life but you could have got yourself into serious trouble."

You ask about an enjoyable experience? (She sat up suddenly and almost rubbed her eyes). My enjoyable experience in nursing was when I was able to move from point A to point B. Suddenly I could advance myself without the restrictions that were throttling me in South Africa. Suddenly I could stand up to my colleagues and say what I wanted without fear of being rapped on the knuckles. It was simply wonderful to work without "white superiority" hanging like a sword of Damocles over my head. Freedom of speech was a most enjoyable, indeed a liberating experience (she paused, and in the silence that followed one could sense the rising emotion. Something akin to illumination shone in her eyes.)

Yes, I experienced crises. In Zambia there were many. I had come from England with all the specialised tertiary care, yet in Zambia you were thrown in at the deep end, having to do literally everything. On duty you had doctors around you from 9-5 but when they went off at 5 – usually to play golf – any emergency that arose after that was *your* problem until the night shift started. There was one doctor on call but the bulk of the work was left in your hands from treating malaria through to gynae and paediatric problems, everything.

I remember sitting in the tearoom once with a colleague, when word came that I had an admission – "a roasted woman" from one of the outlying areas. I thought she was kidding but the patient was "roasted" indeed. Her husband had poured paraffin over her and had set her alight. I absolutely cannot describe the horror of her appearance, the stench of burnt human flesh getting into your nostrils, clothes and everything you eat or touch.

In a state of numb shock I carried out the admission procedure, including the putting up of a drip. In fact I had been taught to put up intravenous infusions by auxiliary nurses. I had humbled myself to them when I first arrived in Zambia, had said, "I do not know how to do this" and they had taught me how. So on this day I was able to handle the severe burns case but unfortunately we were only able to keep her alive for 10 days before she slipped off her mortal coil.

There were frequent occurrences of mining accidents, where we had to go underground to attend to the casualties. One tragic incident, which had me off my moorings for a long time, was when a friend of mine went down one day in the course of duty. While there a further disaster occurred and my friend never came back. I shall never forget that day when the news came through. I had felt as though a block of ice had slipped down my backbone. It was a moment of unbelief. For me her loss is simply endless.

That was the time when there was a war in Zimbabwe the former Rhodesia. People in Zambia suffered the effects of that war especially with regard to food scarcity. Times were very difficult for them, the economic upheavals grave. I had the dichotomous feeling of having job satisfaction but it was tinged with an indescribable sadness, having to watch children suffer from severe malnutrition, having to witness the death of people through starvation. The need for job satisfaction paled into insignificance against this stark reality.

What was especially difficult to cope with on the personal front was the fact that the ex-patriots were treated far better than the Zambians. Reasoning this out was like cracking a tantalising puzzle. I concluded that the contracts were made more attractive so that we could come in and work there. And even though there were such glaring discrepancies I found the Zambians a very humble nation.

There was no bitterness. It's absolutely mind-boggling. Unlike me, who had so much bitterness towards the South African nursing authorities, the Zambian girls taught me a lesson. They taught me an awful lot and I owe them a debt of gratitude for that. It was almost painful to witness how they struggled.

Zambians would go out and queue the whole day for a loaf of bread. It kindled sorrow in the soul. We ex-patriots did not have to do that; we were properly fed. Yet those girls came and worked with us and they worked much harder too and not a frisson of conflict crept in. There were times when I was overcome by an inconsolable melancholy.

Gender problems takes me to England. When I was doing a course in mental nurse training (psychiatry) it was a male-dominated field (her face carries an expression of dogged resistance). Most of them were foreign male nurses from countries like Ireland and Mauritania. There was then simply no scope of advance for a female, the situation being overwhelmed by males. For this reason I left the psychiatric field and went straight into a diploma course in health visiting.

I was intolerant of oppressive situations because of my background. So sharp was my awareness that I was almost paranoid when I came within a whisker of oppression. I had, to a certain extent, paranoia of the white race and its domination.

There was no upward mobility in South Africa where we were kept as "staff-nurses" which made us glorified servants of the whites. Even if you were running a ward as I was in casualty where day-surgery was done in the department and patients where left to recover. I was running that recovery ward but I was supervised by a white. I found that untenable because she did everything she possibly could to interfere in everything I did as a registered nurse. She had her own ward but was as cunning as a weasel and kept her finger in the pie on the black side.

ELLA

As far as difficulties in nursing are concerned, yes there were certainly difficulties, mainly concerning the race factor, which this country is so obsessed with. I had personal difficulties with the fact that you could only be seen in terms of race, that is previously. I say previously because today these things are clouded.

The fact that you were not paid the same salary; you were not regarded nor promoted, all because of the colour of your skin. People these days are promoted to figurehead status and here and there a black face appears in management and people are able to use equal educational opportunities in tertiary studies but on the whole there is still discrimination on the basis of race even today, and for me that is a problem.

I'd like to touch on a professional crisis, which affected me indirectly. This occurred in East London in the psychiatric service, without a CPN (chief professional nurse). Our group was comprised of SPN's (senior professional nurses), PN's and so on. We were then managed by an administration body in Queenstown.

This situation gave rise to an abysmal power-struggle, which brought the person put in charge of us into hateful conflict situations, where this actually spilled over. This is something I would not like to ever have to live through again. It became a vendetta against the person in charge.

Eventually head office – then Pretoria – was called in to sort it out. Our days were marred by the mundane horror of this vendetta. As a result of Pretoria's intervention, the person in charge was demoted, never to be able to rise through the ranks again.

The person who spearheaded this process of demotion was then put in charge of the team until a more senior person was appointed. Amongst our selves this cooked up a storm. In fact, it left such a bitter taste in my mouth that the after-effects are with me still, where I cannot completely trust the system of management in a hierarchy. You don't see them, you don't interact with them, you don't hear what is being discussed, you don't see facts; things simply are not out in the open honestly. The odds are clandestinely banked up against you in heaps.

It can actually be quite frightening when you are suddenly found to be in disfavour and you do not know that until the climax, when you are confronted. I can't remember the exact year when this occurred but it was at the time of the so-called "new dispensation" when promotion became a far-fetched dream and the proffered consolation to nurses was that they could function as senior sisters with the designation of professional nurses. We could not move up from senior sister to senior professional nurse. The impact of this decision on one's career and one's self-esteem was extreme.

RITA

I cannot remember having faced any crisis, no big accidents. The turmoil of 1976 I fortunately missed having been away on leave. But difficulties arose often especially since nursing often seems to contradict itself.

LAHLEKILE

A colleague of mine was recently discussing the ordeal of having to do practicals for tertiary education exams. The fact that one is exposed to ill treatment at the hand of your own colleagues is an astounding truth. You find personnel-in-charge not appreciating what you are doing. Their attitude is: Have you come to work or to study? This is a preposterous line of thinking.

After completing the BA CUR a friend and I went to the nursing service manager's office to inform her of our achievement. This fellow-oppressed sister-in-struggle said nothing, not even the simple word "congratulations." Her silence was somehow dismissive. Uncertainty puckered her face.

Afterwards she went along asking colleagues in her peer group in whispers: "I understand so-and-so has passed. What curriculum is it that they have passed?" Instead of coming to us directly she felt puffed, instead initiating pressure against us.

Another common remark that can hit you in the face is: "I don't care for people with salads on their shoulders." This refers to the qualifications marked by different coloured bars across the epaulettes.

It is incredible that black matrons are capable of passing such derogatory remarks. Their attitude aims to erode the prestige built up by academic achievement. There is neither appreciation nor pride for what we have done. Yet when one embarks on tertiary education one has to surmount tremendous challenges. Many fall by the wayside. What is needed – and I say this in all seriousness – is a bit of star quality bestowed on all those tertiary education students who succeed despite the odds.

These matrons with the negative attitudes started off as nurses with Standard VI who only subsequently managed to reach JC. That is why they do not have insight into nursing education. They are amongst those who oppress their subordinates and who are unable to change.

If they had any kind of dynamism they would have secured posts at the vortex of the power machine but none of them reached Pretoria. None of them did anything to prevent whites from colonising the profession. Fortunately time is phasing them out. Retirement will be the only honourable way out for them.

ESMÉ

There was one tremendous difficulty soon after I qualified. I've never before worked in an Intensive Care Unit and at Grottes you only work there if you are a sister. Qualified staff work in I.C.U. for one week on day duty and one week on night duty.

As soon as the final examination results came out that December, I was immediately designated a sister, not a staff nurse. With immediate effect I was put on duty in the medical respiratory ICU on an 8:5 shift. This was too much for me to handle. I tell you I was scared and went to the matron to explain to her my feeling of total inadequacy. What if anything went wrong? I simply felt ill equipped to handle such a crisis situation as intensive care.

But the matron did not actually want to understand. After I'd been to her office for the third time with still no joy, I went straight over to Maternity and requested that I start middle in January instead of in February, as planned. They accepted me and I was able to retreat from the threatening situation at Grottes.

NOMAMOBALI

The most tremendous stumbling blocks were the matrons, some of whom were nuns, who made life exceedingly unpleasant for us. Imagine a white nun! It seemed as though aliens had invaded our planet specifically to oppress us. Those people were not straight because "straight" is not a term applicable to them in nursing. They were over-strict, over-pressurising us, and we had to train under them.

I've been emotionally scarred by a particularly nasty experience in their hands. It happened on a Sunday afternoon when calamity occurred after a soccer match in Soweto between Kaiser Chiefs and Orlando Pirates. Soccer matches between these two rival soccer factions are rarely peaceful events.

The problem is that both sides have fans and the rivalry is fierce. Kaiser Chiefs wear black and gold and Orlando Pirates black and white. You may go there innocently wearing black and gold, then you are taken as a Kaiser Chief fan. You could be beaten to pulp or trampled upon or even killed.

I was only a novice then, had never seen a corpse in my life and was shaken up at the number of dead and injured arriving on our doorstep. Moreover I was mortified to hear an instruction that I was to lay out those corpses, being of junior status.

Bolting like a rabbit confronted by a fox I locked myself in the toilet and burst into tears. All the while I heard them prowling, hunting me down relentlessly. They shouted: "Where is the junior nurse?" They did not even know my name. One said gleefully: "Today she is going to shit bricks!"…[This is how I interpreted her Sotho]….."Today she is going to lay out those corpses for she is the most junior nurse."

Another experience indelibly scorched on my mind is my sojourn in the operating theatre while still a junior. I stood out like a sore thumb for being the one with the least skills. One day all the trained staff were occupied in the theatre and there came an emergency case where I happened to be. A nightmare situation unfolded for me when the surgeons made a lightening decision that open-heart surgery had to be done immediately.

I was in a total daze when they called upon me to scrub, regardless of the fact that I did not know one instrument from the other. I was totally in the dark too about what to do and what not to do. Altogether a terrifying situation.

Throughout the operation we were standing on our feet, something quite tortuous to the novice. Imagine open-heart surgery from 8pm to the following day! Unlike birth pains, soon-to-be-forgotten, I shall remember the unbearable ache in my feet to my last day on earth, and what they looked like afterwards. Well-risen dough is the best way that I can describe those feet.

LAHLEKILE

When at last it was over, I made my way directly to the matron's office. In fact I handed in my resignation through a mist of tears. The sister (at Bara the sisters act as secretaries to the matron) said to me: "There is no way that you are going to up and leave in this manner. You are going to stay in nursing."

I felt throttled. An enormous lump arose in my throat, which I could hardly swallow over. They were pressurising me to become something my spirit was rebelling against. The feeling that I did not want to be a nurse threatened to overwhelm me. Even today as I'm sitting here, I still reject this occupation because there have been too many negative experiences which I could have done without.

The patients I remember vividly were three children, one a little boy who was a cardiac sufferer, another little boy with nephritis and a diabetic girl with a colostomy. The three of them stole my heart with their ability to sing. We used to sing together. One child could sing "Teba ka mo" which means "to guard." He sang this in a clear, ringing voice, which carried like a bell and he would dramatise the words with actions, how he was guarding things well. Often I tasted the salt of my own tears, knowing how short his life was likely to be.

One day I went to town and bought – for their delight – chips, sweets and peanuts, only to discover that I had forgotten the condition of their illnesses. One child could not eat peanuts, another sweets; in the end the planned surprise melted swiftly away with me guzzling tearfully, all by myself in my room. To this day I have their photograph and their memory never fails to wrap me in a cloud of melancholia.

I faced a professional crisis of huge dimensions right at the start with the Soweto riots in 1976 when school children defied the state over the introduction of Afrikaans as a compulsory language. I think it was Dr Andries Treurnicht who did that.

Anyway, we at Bara could not leave the hospital premises because of the stone throwing and the frenzy of violence that was spreading through the township like wild fire through dry grass. Besides, we were bound for duty at the casualty department. That was when I learned to deal with a crisis because we were led into a pattern of action. Still, it was most terrible.

We were unable to differentiate between male and female patients, so covered in blood were those children. Their clothes were torn and parts of their bodies shot off. And the tear gas effect was simply unbelievable. If their skins had been white, there would have been total pandemonium. White parents would have jerked out of control, I'm sure.

The deaths were something else. Before our very eyes, the children simply died like flies. We nurses literally jumped over their corpses like toads over river rocks, attending urgently to those who showed a breath of life. Across Soweto, all we could see was voluminous black smoke clogging the sky.

In fact the situation in Soweto at that time was simply venomous. We could not spare a second to think of ourselves. Much as I wanted to make a professional U-turn, it was not possible to do so at a time when young people were dying as easily as we were breathing.

LAHLEKILE

I recall one student, said to be very bright, whose sister was training with us. Apparently she was unaware that she had been deserted by her peers at the time when they came directly into the firing line of the police. In fact they were shot at. Somehow, inexplicably, she had found that those she had been with, had withdrawn without her. They seem to have acted according to a different set of imperatives.

Today that beautiful young lady spends her life in a wheelchair. I read in a newspaper that she had joined Mabuse and Co. but the tragedy hits me, because she was known to be intellectually superior, having outstanding good looks besides.

Really, that riot was a time when you concentrated totally on helping others to survive their injuries. I remember how we talked in disconnected sentences while we worked. The hospital resembled a battlefield. The Battle of Trafalgar could not have been worse.

Behind the situation one struggled with impressions and impulses one could neither relate nor control. You worked remorselessly, driven to the brink of hysteria. All in all the loss of life was enormous.

One thought will always niggle. Will the perpetrators of this violence - not the state itself, which is ultimately responsible, but the young men who carried out the orders – will they or their children escape scot-free from the bloody deeds of Soweto 1976?

As for "difficulties" in nursing…you tempt my brain to sing a bitter litany. Yes, I had lots of difficulties, even up to today. High on the list is the communication problems.

During training days the supervisors were all white. As far as I'm concerned they were as emotional as snails, clinging to their desks like leeches. Each time you went there with a burning problem, first you had to have permission. You felt like a criminal attempting to pass through the hands of customs officials. As far as your problems were concerned, these people were unapproachable because they had no idea of you as a person.

A communication problem as impenetrable as the Berlin Wall lay between them and us. I had the ringing impression that they simply did not see blacks as human beings but as a work package, which they listed as a unit of labour. A good example of "man's inhumanity to man" don't you think? They seemed to have devised an artificial way of thinking and behaving in their interactions with us.

Nowadays in 1992, with the NEW SOUTH AFRICA splashed all over the mass media, I'm still living in the "old" South Africa. Could anyone indicate please, where is the new? Unless something drastic happens, I don't think that I shall be staying in the profession for much longer. I am not going to doom myself to a life of emptiness, servility and suppressed misery.

Working in the operating theatre is another form of hell. This is an area where tensions naturally bubble to the surface and for me the outstanding feature about the theatre situation was the rudeness of the whites in charge, most particularly the doctors.

LAHLEKILE

When I first came to the Eastern Cape I agitated for a meeting so that I could air my grievances. Not that this got me anywhere, not with the bureaucratic grievance procedure, which is more confusing than helpful.

These doctors would catapult themselves through the theatre doors with effusive greetings for the white and coloured nurses. They would say, "Good morning Nurse so-and-so…." Meanwhile you were standing there with a tray in readiness and this doctor did not choose to recognise your presence, did not even bother to know your name. Tell me please, who is a better person, the one who scrubs up and snubs you, or the one who is the "hewer of wood and drawer of water" in the theatre?

To show their complete disdain for a black professional nurse, these doctors had bantering jokes together, drawing the white nurses in under a river of recognition. They would chat to one another: "How is your child? I understand your child is ill?" "Oh, I've bought the latest TV game for my child…." And dare you come up to them for whatever reason, as a black nurse, their faces become masses of sheer rock. They will say: "Give me this" or "Give me that" and it all ends there.

I was intensely interested in theatre work but the attitude of doctors thoroughly discouraged me. A doctor can change into an angry beast just because he finds himself next to a black skin. And its not only the doctors, mind.

A colleague told us how they were busy putting a patient under anaesthesia one day. A white nurse came up to the patient and said: "Why are you looking so anxious? Is it because there are so many black skins around that you cannot fall asleep?" She swears those were the actual words and there was no evidence that the nurse was clowning.

I had a similar experience when a patient said to me, as she was about to go under, "I shouldn't like to have a black nurse next to me when I wake up." And I can tell you that her voice was entirely devoid of remorse.

I have not had upward mobility. I have not gone up anywhere and I don't think it is an option for me unless, unless, unless…it all changes.

There are countless colleagues of mine who have got degrees, some more than one, and they have gone nowhere with academic excellence. Like packs of hungry wolfhounds we are all jostling at the bottom rung of the ladder, all professional nurses. Postgraduate qualifications are conveniently ignored. Not so with the white nurses, many of them end up with diplomas rather than degrees.

All you need to be in nursing is white and then the sky is the limit for you. They are up there as chief professional nurses, nursing organisers, nursing service managers, standing above us like poles above water. I pray for the black nurses who pursue academic excellence despite everything. I admire them for their perseverance in the face of the low position in the hierarchy. Things might change for them.

A thought has just struck me. Look at the nurses around us, all in white dresses and some having honours degrees. Then look at the nursing service managers strutting around in their special uniforms of colour. They do not walk without a measure of arrogance. I am struck by the injustice of the situation, the downright dishonesty of the system. That is one of the things being done to oppress us.

I have not had gender problems with male nurses, but of course with doctors and I'd like to amplify my observations. They would not treat their wives, girl friends, nor any white woman the way they treat us. They dehumanise us, not merely by not greeting or not knowing our names, but by ignoring our professional status and by taking us as their maids in the wards. Even now in the nineties, here in the Cape, I have never encountered so many rude doctors.

When I was in training at Baragwanath, at the end of each month when there was a changeover, the doctors used to buy cake and share it with the nurses who so faithfully assisted them in their work. But here, I should imagine the overwhelming number of doctors to be products of the *AWB, because they display such indifference and open rudeness to blacks, its as though they suffer a kind of xenophobia as far as we are concerned.

Officially the book on apartheid has been closed. Yet in nursing we still belong to that era of "Yes matron…no matron…so sorry matron…" These words are thorns in the throat but we parrot them nevertheless. To us, apartheid is a bottomless sea. The entire image of nursing needs to be changed. Black nurses have been oppressed for so long that they still willingly follow white nurses like puppets on a string. Even if the white nurse is doing something wrong, the black nurse will in most cases back away, not wanting to be part of an impending show-down. The white nurse is "the boss".

I should think that this is the time for us to change things. We cannot wait for the time when we know that the hard logic of arithmetic will assess itself in South African nursing, in fact in the entire economic structure as it must.

Historically, whenever great change occurs in society there is always great upheaval to the point of war. But all we ask for in nursing is for the profession to become acceptable to the space age. We want nursing to emerge from its cocoon of traditional attitudes of oppression of blacks and we want that to happen now.

Many of the nurses were furious at having wasted their time. I naturally felt emotionally abused too. I believe that the black nurses must stop being so polite. We should begin to unsheathe our claws ever so good-naturedly. The rights of nurses have got to be addressed at higher levels right into the Nursing Act.

This can be done if we stretch the web of democracy extensively enough.

* Afrikaner Resistance Movement

MAGDALENA

I still shudder to think of all the corpses we had to handle. Those dead bodies were simply horrifying to me. The absolute last straw was when a bad experience sent me charging like a bat out of the attic.

It happened when I was working in Casualty. There was a patient with a back deformity who suffered cardiac arrest. Every effort was made to resuscitate him but still, he died. We juniors, who had to deal with his remains, were confronted by an unusual problem; we simply could not get the body to stay down. My eyes exploded from my head when the body suddenly sprang up into a sitting position. I don't remember that my feet touched the ground when I ran. Some of the nurses went into hysterics, even the sisters got hiccups bottling their laughter.

But I remember some very pathetic cases too, especially the one in which a fat patient died. A younger doctor put her up on a drip at Maternity. When I saw him pumping fluids into her I asked him what he thought he was doing? He replied that he was "re-hydrating" her. I disagreed with this treatment and told him so. It seemed that I'd put my head in the lion's jaw by daring to express an opinion.

She was a mother of ten and her death was a hard pill for me to swallow. His stereotypical response was "Who-do-you-think-you-are" but I let him have a bit of my mind. In fact we landed up in the matron's office after I allowed myself a little freedom of language in berating him.

I learned then that a nurse's word does not carry any weight. And you can't go far in exposing this type of malpractice either. Even up to today medicine is mostly for whites as few of us can make it. The system looks after it's own. This was a young inexperienced white doctor.

Another thing that I found frightening in Cape Town – though the general population is very nice – was the great number of schizophrenics who attended the Avalon Centre near the Nico Malan College.

I was scared out of my scull to see on the same disco floor as ourselves, striking young men, lithe and handsome, but *we* knew that they were jam-packed with every neurosis in the book. The thought of an inevitable personal catastrophe was so frightening that I made up my mind to keep off the dating scene while in Cape Town.

But the people of Cape Town on the whole are extremely nice. I quite enjoyed nursing the people and interacting with them. None of my grouses were concerned with patients. In fact it was precisely because of the patients that I managed to hang on in nursing long after my family's finances were out of the doldrums. I especially liked the up-country folk who exuded an air of simplicity and trust. What a tragedy that their lives have become compounded by mass rural poverty as a result of apartheid turning the countryside into catchment areas for surplus (black) population.

My difficulties were – and still are – with the hours, with night duty and with the fact that nursing is so totally dominated by doctor's orders. Some of these doctors, especially the novices, can be such pricks, both as doctors and as people, and they feel threatened by us. Their meanness at times and their will to exploit, these have become ingrained cultural reflexes.

LAHLEKILE

Then at Frere in the Eastern Cape the black-white situation is bad. There the atmosphere is beset by a maze of crosscurrents. It was a shock to find when I started there that the terrible "boertjie" matrons were so insistent on doing things the old-fashioned way, like dressings, for instance. It was hard for me to have to step down from a good teaching hospital like "Grottes" to one where obsolescence prevails.

Suddenly you had to do your own packs - this in the eighties – and all those old-fashioned dressings, everything hopelessly outdated, including the attitudes which are totally unacceptable in an enlightened era.

One is happy to note that the situation is changing numerically. The whites are not coming into nursing so much. Maybe those who do are filled with saccharine ideals or relieving boredom or for whatever reason, but we come into the profession because of necessity. If we don't work we starve and so the numbers are weighted in favour of blacks despite the meticulous attention paid to skewing the intake on racial lines.

Whereas in the past they would not want black staff touching a white on a bed, things have changed through sheer lack of staff of the required colour. We're in the majority now and they're in a fix, they need nurses.

As far as I know, nursing has always been inundated with double standards. Like the classical case at Frere Maternity where up to the recent eighties you, as a black person, were not allowed to set foot in their theatre except when they were in a fix, then suddenly it became okay for you to do so.

But Blacks are coming into their own today, well able through political enlightenment to escape the bondage in which they were held. And the whites have not learned to cope with that yet. They're so used to being the masters and us the willing slaves, that they remain suspicious even today.

Blacks are becoming much better qualified and we're willing to work the hours. Yet even in my present position – and we've hit the nineties – where I work in a private institution, the doctors who own the place are forever getting some white to come in part-time to come and help them out, to run things for them.

After a few months such a nurse will pack up and take flight, being very suspicious of the polyglot environment starting up. That is how things are. It will take light-years for the myth of white supremacy to be scorched to ashes.

There was one enjoyable experience, but it was not directly concerned with nursing. I went to work in the United States of America for a year and a bit and came home when my father passed away.

The American experience was a fun situation for me. My emotions began to curve skywards. The poor American nurses are under so much pressure because of all the potential lawsuits they might encounter.

Nursing there was a novel experience in that those patients could almost worship us South African nurses. We were found to be hard working, contrary to here (broad mischievous smile) where you're constantly berated for being "slap." There we were able to take the initiative to instigate some humane actions. I don't know why in South Africa you get no credit even if you do your level best. Here the doctors often show resentment if you do well in Casualty but in the U.S.A. they express their appreciation. By the way, the other nurses who worked really hard were the Irish girls. They work like donkeys.

There was no enjoyable situation in nursing in this country. I was always miserable, always hungry too, a famished wolfhound, forever eating the patients' delicacies, which was not really permissible.

One of the reasons why nursing lacks joy is because there's not enough participation from the grassroots level. No input is required of students or professional nurses, who are merely the mules pulling the cart, and the very idea of the ethos of nursing as propounded by South African authors, is repugnant to me. The total submission that is required of you is completely abhorrent.

Nursing is a very narrow world run by narrow people. Those in charge pontificate from the heights of white authority. And those even higher up continue waffling on and on about the noble spirit of nursing but their message is falling on stony ground.

The ethos of nursing aims to focus attention on patient needs above all else. But what it does in a kind of subterranean manner is to calculatedly crush the individual's verve and spirit.

After a stint of nursing things change for you. You become afraid to venture out as a self-assured person.

That's what nursing does to you, it kills the motivation and its not really strange that you have a lot of cheque collectors these days, because nurses are not required to give any meaningful creative input, at the level that you are able to do this. That is not encouraged.

For example, what the doctor says goes. This tenet is a bit ridiculous; in fact I find it traumatic that doctors should be so elevated. Why? After all, they are doing their job at *their* level and we are doing ours at *our* level. In-between, society has to cope with the side effects as best it can.

So why look down upon nurses as much as they do? Why do nurses always have to present as a picture of prudence? As much as they are elevated we are trampled in the dust. Automatically the doctors do not acknowledge black nurses and I find that such a problem. Even today, in the nineties, there is so much *talk* about change but at grassroots level the situation remains the same. This is something, which hurts the mind.

I'm not out to crucify doctors, but in the here and now of it, nurses experience the situation in most hospitals as I've described. The doctor has a heart as impenetrable as a nutmeg.

I have faced countless professional crises in the course of duty, especially in casualty, where nurses have to make split-second decisions when a doctor happens not to be there.

One day a patient fell off a theatre table because there was no one to attend to him. He fractured his scull in the fall. There happened to be no doctor around for this emergency. I sutured with shaky fingers, and gave a shot of Bicillin, all without doctors. Nurses simply do what has to be done, and get their actions verified afterwards. They take risks and sometimes do not have a leg to stand on.

In I.C.U. there is a different scenario. Here too, you do whatever is necessary under emergency conditions and far too often when doctors are not on the spot, nurses are left to plug the gap.

For one thing, even before you call the doctor you must have the venal lines open and by this means alone you save many lives. Many patients I've helped in this way have recovered. I've seen them walking around afterwards, alive and well. But nowhere is it recognised what the nurse has done, even if her nursing expertise is stretched beyond her limit, especially then.

In cases where only a thread of life remains, it is the nurse who at times has to do the resuscitation, the defib, stuff like that. You work while neon lights flash in your head. These are gritty and realistic aspects of nursing.

In a six-bedded I.C.U. there is only one registered nurse and two E.N.A's (enrolled nursing assistants). As the sister you are responsible for writing up the nursing process. Furthermore, your duties include doing E.C.G's, taking bloods – sometimes from the tiniest veins, Intravenous therapy and the like. The IV therapy may be four-hourly and then it's your responsibility to see that every drop goes in every four hours.

Then there are airstrips, part of blood chemistry, "listening" to the patients' fears. It's a totally different set-up for the patient to be in I.C.U., quite terrifying one can imagine and the nurse has to be more explicit in her communication. She plays a major psychological role to reassure patients who often are too ill to communicate their fears.

The work is energy sapping for a nurse. All that the E.N.A's do is back-and-pressure parts. Their vision ends with the crisp rustle of clean sheets. Everything else is left to the nurse. For instance, if a patient does not pass urine, you are left with the problem of how to or get the patient to pee otherwise they could go into renal failure, or toxaemia. You assess all the time and it can be profoundly stressful.

The responsibility of having to prevent someone from going into renal failure is a good illustration of the strain the nurse is under because on top of those lifesaving decisions she has to make, she's bogged down by more and more work and the next day, starchy Florence Nightingales drift along to ask a lot of crap – why hasn't a suction tube been changed? Forgetting that she's had the strain of having to keep six people alive. In that respect things simply must change.

EUCLID

My main difficulty was with the hours, especially weekends. I dodged around the weekend shift so much that it nearly cost me my career. A feeling of martyrdom set in. I had to stop partaking in sport, my training programmes had to be ruthlessly scissored out of my life, something that I found devastating. Nursing really curbed my lifestyle. I still don't know what kept me going.

The off-duties were the bone of contention in my life.

Reduced weekends I wanted to be home, that was the bottom line. I was prepared to resort to bribery for that. During weekend duty you work in a daze. In a way you need to be in a daze, otherwise the sheer terror of your social dislocation could overwhelm you and get you to throw in the towel.

Night duty was no less terrible. I still cannot get used to it even now that my mind is more focussed. During student days it made me feel that the top of my head was going to blow off. Each time I faced night duty my stomach either began to run under relentless peristaltic command or it cramped with spasms.

It's not the work itself, because once I'm there the work is no big deal, I can devour work. It is the psychological set-up of having to go to work at night. That puts one off course. I get queasy just thinking about it. Day duty on the other hand is perfectly fine because then one has a little time to spend with one's self and one's family.

There were problems too as far as interpersonal relationship were concerned. There were all those vocal remorseless matrons with signs of obsolescence, and there were a few sisters who tried to emulate them.

I shudder to think what those sisters are like today for some of them are still occupying posts, those who spoke in tones that brooked no rejoinders. If they were outdated then, I wouldn't want to know what they are like now.

Anyway I had my close encounters with these people. I remember on one occasion when a vacolitre had to be changed. This sister could not make out what the doctor's order was yet she would not allow me to proceed to put up the vac. Her attitude was puzzling for I was able-bodied and qualified and perfectly able to read the instructions while she was unable to see what she was about. She actually forbade me to touch the drip until she returned.

I thought in some astonishment that she had gone to the telephone the doctor to reaffirm what he had prescribed but in fact she had gone to the duty room to fetch her spectacles. She said she could not allow a "blue junior" like me to do anything without her confirming my actions.

She found that what I had read was correct and we put up the vacolitre. However, our relationship took a bad turn because I felt that trust had been broken. That was one isolated case.

The point that I'm making is that obsolescence on the part of older staff played a negative role in my nursing education.

I have not had an enjoyable experience, I'd be lying if I told you I had one. Man, nursing is just generally a miserable life. But if I could quote the memorable times I spent in nursing then I'd have to mention Casualty.

LAHLEKILE

In Casualty one reels continuously from one disastrous case to another. It puts one in mind of what Nietzsche called "the eternal wound of being."

Many patients there are stunned out of their minds – the drunken dissolute weekend alcoholics, the Blacks who get crushed by sledgehammer violence, the Coloureds who get stabbed, the occasional rape cases which come in – it seemed that the clinical set-up with its simple technological tools, was the backcloth for the human stories enacted in the foreground.

You moved in and around the tragedies, taking histories from distraught people and somehow you made your own moments pleasant, often laughing spontaneously when you heard the ludicrous tales of how people got into their situations. For example, an incongruous figure in a dinner jacket does not want to be identified because he came in at 4am having had an accident. When you want to call his next of kin he says, in a rigid defensive posture with a wavering desperation in his eyes: "No, no, please. I'll do that myself."

It was an intriguing task having to put telling anecdotes into concrete terms, often shaking with laughter in the process. And the smell in Casualty could often be overpowering. You dealt with scores of people day after day, at least a thousand over a weekend, and they were all unique. Casualty had an implacable rhythm. There was always humour.

A professional crisis hit me way back in 1985. There was all of a sudden a mass uprising of black students. This volatile confrontation between the youth and the state was enticing the youth to fraternal suicide…

I was in charge of the Frere Casualty and was suddenly confronted by very serious choices, which threw me out on a limb. I had to be loyal to my Employing Body; had to dig into my inner reserves to find the quality of humanness needed in the caring aspect of nursing, but what about my loyalty to the people, to the forces of liberation? Some of them had been brutally abused in an atrocious and revolting way.

It was a terrifying experience. Soon it became apparent that patients needed to stay away from hospital territory because of the danger of being followed there by police with uncompromising attitudes who arrested them on trolleys, for public violence and intimidation. Truly I was in a spiral of black despair.

I was an asset to the medical personnel fresh off the campus and taught countless numbers of them diagnostic and therapeutic procedures. It amused me to notice their young faces when presented with strange phenomena such as perhaps a skin eruption unfamiliar to them. They'd have inscrutable countenances but you could see that their minds were straining at the lcash. "Oh, but this is a funny rash" they'd say. When I'd point out that it was "shingles", knowing that they could not recognise it, they'd cry: "How do you know?" And I'd toss out a careless: "Well I've seen enough of it."

One day a lady doctor met me in town and was so overcome with impulsive joy that she hugged me right there on the pavement in Oxford Street. "Euclid how are you?" she exclaimed, in a voice warm with emotion. Turning to her doctor friends, she proudly announced: "This is Euclid. In Casualty he taught me how to do a ring block." They were surprised, more I think, because human kindness and friendship is not a commodity that is easily passed between black and white.

At another time I nearly overstepped my scope of practice when I snatched a scalpel from a doctor's lifeless hand and showed her where to put it in to make an emergency tracheotomy.

The patient was having great difficulty in breathing and was going to die and she stood there shivering with fright. I mustered military tones: "Get the patient straight, do this, do that, get the knife in here. I actually pressed her hand to commence the cut. She did not know what to do with the tube so I yelled, "Put the tube in here" in staccato tones and guided her once again. Mercifully the patient survived. She went outside and cried but came afterwards to say "Thank you Euclid." I felt pity for her but had to take a stern line.

Some patients actually came after their recovery to express gratitude and that is the finest compliment that can be made. One day a hothead novice discarded the idea of suturing a partly severed ear, which was dangling on a piece of skin. "Ag, it will never take", he said, exuding an aura of defeat. "Now what have you got to lose? If the ear doesn't take, then so what? At least we would have tried." But he shrugged indifferently and left.

I tried raising Mr R the plastic surgeon but he wouldn't come out and we were running out of time. So I scrubbed the ear, scrubbed the surface. It took me three-and-a-half hours to suture the ear back. I had to suture inside the canal as well, very fine suturing with 60 nylon, inside the ear. It worked!

The next evening I went to the ward to remove the dressing. Sure enough, the ear was there, sitting safe. I removed the plug of gelignite. The nurses had no idea what was in the ear. A few days later I removed the stitches too. I then showed this to the reluctant doctor who was considerably impressed.

JOY

The most difficult time of all was 1992. There was a strike arranged by NEHAWU. We in the labour ward, utterly in the grip of nerves, decided not to go out. All the other nurses had gone, leaving paediatrics lying in wards etc. unattended. We in the labour wards were then expected to fill in those departments, something that threw us on the horns of a dilemma.

The chief matron descended on us with a massive verbal lashing, thereby greatly underrating our stand. We had in fact taken a risk in not going out on strike. If we stood in for those who had gone out it would have appeared as though we were undermining their cause.

With a sour grunt the matron said, "Show me one person here who applied for a post in the labour ward." There was no gainsaying her argument. I felt myself trembling from the whole aggressive atmosphere. She wanted us to spread the manpower yet we would be putting our heads on the chopping block and risking the lives of our families too, not to mention the burning down of our houses.

LAHLEKILE

I shall never forget the agony of indecision, which befell us. It hurt even more since our intentions were of the best. We had to weigh everything up with such intensity I thought my eyes would pop out of my head. We looked at our lives with a strange detachment, almost like spectators.

In the end we walked out and joined the strike leaving behind us patients in the various stages of labour. That was the most dispiriting part of all. I felt that day like crawling into a hole like a wounded animal and staying there forever.

FLO

As for crisis situations, well I had one hell of a crisis after my second Block at Tygerberg, on night duty. I was in charge of a busy block with the sister covering three wards. I had one other student to assist me in the surgical ward. We received a patient from theatre who died virtually on arrival at the ward. We were almost taken to court because of that case.

The matron marched in and stated so brashly my hair stood stiff: "I want to find out who murdered this patient," she said. To my alarm, the sister seemed struck dumb and was unable to inform her concisely of the situation under which we had worked.

I then raised my voice to ask whether she had investigated the patient's history, surgical intervention and his prognosis; whether she had investigated what part we had played in all this, and what circumstances we had worked under?

That saved the day for us. I even found the courage to say: "I object to your choice of words; to your treatment of us; to the way you allocate your staff. We did what we could but we could not decide when people had to die."

Something good came out of that tirade. We got an extra nurse on night duty. I could not accept that the chief matron could conduct an enquiry in that manner. It was an outrage!

AUDREY

I had difficulty at the start of my career when I could not get a post in a hospital so I accepted employment from a private practitioner. I would see patients over a 24-hour service because the people would come at any time, day or night. I was too timid to complain since it had taken me a long time to secure the job. All my applications had backfired with regret...regret...regret. So I had the advantage of learning primary health care under the doctor who taught me how to use the stethoscope.

In that area (Seymour) I had to be sure that the patients were not faking. There had been a spasm of protest at my appointment because I hailed from the Transkei and they grumbled too because the doctor allowed a nurse to examine them. I really feared at times that their sole reason for coming to the doctor's surgery was to attack me. It was my good fortune that Seymour was largely in a coma by night.

Most of the time I was left holding the baby. Often I would end up taking the patient to my home, putting up a drip, observing through the night, but as time went on things straightened out a bit. CPA took over the clinic;

the doctor left for Cape Town. Woefully though, we had to continue working the 24 hour service.

ALFRED

I experienced the difficulty of a conflict situation, black on black, between a ward supervisor and myself. Either everything I did was wrong or she had a faultfinding propensity. She was a woman who was always correct, contained, persistent. She could not allow me to express myself in any way. It was a ludicrous position to be in, always having to keep quiet.

She had a diploma in midwifery and as far as I was concerned she was my senior because of her wealth of practical experience. It is difficult in a one-on-one relationship to say it was because of the glaring gap in qualifications. It might have been a personal dislike.

(Editor's note: On the personal front I found the interviewee to be physically attractive. He exuded a kind of male sexuality that was totally casual from his side. Moreover his voice had a kind of low-key crack in it as though there was an abundance of feeling beneath the surface. It is not inconceivable that females could easily be drawn to him. His body language seemed to proclaim the message I'm – a lazy – tiger).

ALFRED CONTINUES

One can look at a person maybe of the opposite sex and say, "I don't like what I see." That's a cradle-to-grave thing that won't fizzle out. It all sounds devious but it was not. We simply haggled through the time we were forced to share the work situation. I had a friend who was supporting me throughout the ordeal. He said to me, "You have a higher qualification than her and she feels threatened." I didn't want to see it as such. Unlike me he preferred blowing hot air instead of smoking the pipe of peace.

I think what was important for me at that stage was that it is not so much why things happen but what you do when it does. So for me it was more important that I be able to deal with the situation. I knew that the only thing that would float me free was not confrontation but how I did my work. And I had my finger on the button in that regard. And though it was a rotten situation to be in I survived her entrenched chauvinism (a sheepish grin plucks at the corners of his mouth).

FARIEDA

A crisis occurred one day in Durban when a student colleague and I walked smack into a shattering street scene. Those days student nurses were not allowed to wear uniforms in town precisely because when confronted with street accidents they might be at a loss what to do.

On the day that the two of us came upon the accident we were in mufti but I said to my friend, "Look, we're nurses, we cannot stand by and do nothing."

On pressing through the crowd we saw some professional nurses from another hospital standing at a bus stop close by, in tense postures. They too had witnessed the accident but to our astonishment they were not swinging into action to assist the people who were injured. My friend and I looked at each other. For a moment out mouths dropped open though not a sound emerged. I felt anger brewing up inside me. They stood there as though assistance was not within the compass of their imagination. There can be no excuse for this from any point of view.

We focussed our attention on the injured. Two adults were lying in the street tended by a "lay" man who seemed grateful for our assistance. The thought flashed through my mind that this man needed to unload some of his anguish on to someone else.

While my friend looked at one of the injured, I examined another, ascertained that he was conscious and could move his neck and arms, so I decided that we could move him to the pavement. Very worrying though was that I could hear the faint cries of a child. It sent a shimmer of fear skitter up my back for there was no child in sight.

Because our skills were limited my stomach felt as if it had squirrels jumping around inside. The sudden sound of sirens in the distance was soothing as it meant that help was at hand. When the paramedics came I said to them, "There's a child crying somewhere" and they listened but could not hear anything above the noise of the traffic and the crowd milling around. All their attention was focussed on getting the injured adults into the ambulance.

However, when they caught the tone of incipient hysteria in my voice at last I gained their full attention. I could definitely detect the feeble cries of a child, I insisted. So they dove headlong into the recesses of the two cars that had collided, their large, strong hands plunging down to search every inch until at last a little toddler was discovered upside down underneath a back seat where the child had fallen and slipped through.

The child's rescue, which drew a murmur from the crowd, was sweet to my senses, overwhelming to the emotions. I was very excited indeed to have been instrumental in saving that child who was curled into a foetal ball, whimpering from time to time.

We felt elated too, for being ordinary student nurses, now being thanked effusively by the public who were not aware that a group of trained people were standing indifferent to the scene. It left an indelible impression on my mind that the starchy demeanour of some professional nurses can easily melt under heat. I vowed that I should be a different type off nurse.

PETER

Difficulties there certainly were and are. My lack of promotion really bugs me. Even though I was often told that I was doing well, people far less conversant with ward routine somehow always got placed in charge of me. On night duty I excelled to the extent that everything was often left in my hands when I was asked to take over the functional line. I would dilute myself all over the place keeping things running. On countless occasions I'd be sent to Casualty to help out in a crisis, yet no one who mattered bothered to say "Thank you, well done." What they articulated without difficulty was that I was too young to be promoted and that they did not want to offend anybody, that's what I was told. It was palpably unfair and left me feeling flat and helpless.

LAHLEKILE

The other difficulty, which hit me indirectly, was the treatment meted out to Tammy. During my student days she ran the largest ward in the hospital. I first became aware of her qualities during a demonstration in which she role-played the part of a patient, giving a credible performance. In time we became close and what made the earth shake for me was her ability to make me feel special.

She was transferred to the administration block though she was at the level of professional nurse at the time. Four years ago she was rank-promoted to senior professional nurse. This means that you receive the salary but not the designation. Is that not thoroughly demoralising? Her duties are formidable and include allocation of students to the wards, terminations, and appointments. She does things that I am immensely proud of but from a lower rank than she deserves. They turn a blind eye to her competency and care only about her private life, which they sniffed into like hound dogs that cut me to the quick. As far as I'm concerned a person should be promoted according to their competency not their private life, if this is within the ambit of the law. I regard this style of management as dark and claustrophobic and fail to see why our courtship should have raised so much spleen.

My work in I.C.U. deserves comment I think, because of the difficulties experienced there. I practically ran the "black" I.C.U. although there was a sister-in-charge. I organised everything, requisitioning, the trolley, what had to go where. Without any training in this specialised from of nursing I nevertheless innovated wherever I could, like making trolleys more practically useful, changing the dressing room, even getting cupboards installed for vacolitres, the works.

Then I approached the sister-in-charge to request that we arrange in-service training once a week for staff in a teaching-learning experience. Regrettably when I opted out of I.C.U. eventually, everything just fell apart especially after the sister-in-charge had been moved too.

There was a significant occurrence one day when we had to nurse a dying baby whose glucose level was so low that there was a risk of brain damage. We had to get the glucose level raised so that the brain could be fed and kept going. Normally the glucose level should be above 2 but this baby remained at 1,9. The doctor took blood and sent it to the laboratory. I was shocked when the lab report stated that the blood was 54. This was simply incredible.

The doctor was equally surprised when I phoned to tell him and ordered that the intravenous fluids be changed immediately. I said agitatedly, "Doctor before we do that will you let me first check on the other unit's gloconometre? Maybe our apparatus is faulty. When I got the same reading on the other gloconometre we changed the fluid. But something niggled my brain. I phoned the lab and on my own initiative asked the technician to come and do a needle stick. She obliged and promptly phoned the results through. The blood reading was not 54 but 1,4. As it happened, the doctor had just phoned through. There I was with two phones in my hand. When he heard the news he barked, "Change the fluid back to what it was before." He then charged up to the unit, shook my hand and said "Thank you."

LAHLEKILE

As far as administration was concerned, no one indicated to me that I had done anything extraordinary. "It's your job," they said morosely. How can it be my job when I'm working above norm? It was fortunate for the patients that I had somehow acquired a questioning mind and was able to formulate strategies of my own.

Apart from the everyday crises of I.C.U. a potential crisis affected us at the time when the Oceanos liner was sinking off the treacherous Transkei coast. It bothered me that people in I.C.U. seemed unconcerned about taking preparatory action. I took it upon myself to approach the casualty matron to enquire as to why we were not swinging into action. Ten minutes later a doctor came and began to clear the beds for an emergency. The patients who could be moved were sent to the wards.

As it happened we did not get any patients because most of the passengers had been rescued before the ship went down. Casualty received a few cases of hypothermia but they were not unconscious so they did not require intensive care but I felt excited by the event that had shaken up so many lives from across the world.

Crises occur on a daily basis in I.C.U. such as patient's arrests and you have to know what to do, whom to call, how to delegate work to your nurses because there are other patients who need intensive hands-on nursing. It could happen that you are alone with two nurses when a patient arrests. In such an event I should take the most senior of the two to assist me with decisive intervention until the doctor arrives. The other nurse would have to carry on with the rest of the essential abnormalities such as urinary output of less than 50 200mls before we call a doctor to see if that will help? Such grave responsibilities would be carried out by three of us, this on a daily basis and in my case with only three years experience as a qualified nurse.

Gender problems occur with doctors who are uncertain how to handle a male nurse. Nursing was always female dominated and doctors are predominantly male. They tend to regard female black sisters as somehow inferior and do not understand black women in more aggressive or forceful roles.

These days they have to contend with male nurses more and more and of course they cannot regard their own sex as inferior too. So they have problems relating to me and I have problems with them regarding nursing as inferior. I deplore the dual discrimination – doctors versus nurses and white versus black.

Another thing I cannot handle very well is the fact that I have to consult a doctor on every single thing and not make my own decisions because nurses are professionals in their own right. Why does a doctor have to determine how much work I do? He would say "Six hourly" or "Two-hourly" or whatever. Those are really nursing decisions.

There are no problems with female colleagues. On the contrary ladies from the Xhosa culture tend to treat me with great respect, maybe because culturally men are respected. What we need to strive for is a unified non-racial gender-blind health delivery service.

LAHLEKILE

AN INTERNATIONAL EXPERIENCE

DENISE [1983 TRAINEE]

My career as a nursing assistant began nine years ago when I commenced training and then began to work at the big hospital here in Saskatchewan. Presently I have been at a Nursing Home – where I like to be – for the last five years.

Nursing is something that I always wanted to do. When I first went to Canada with my husband, who preferred to live in exile rather than under the yoke of apartheid, I saw that there was a chance for me, because I found myself in a country brimming with opportunities.

In South Africa there was no money for us to go on with schooling beyond the secondary level. In fact I had to go to work very early to help support the family. When I got abroad I said "well now, let's see if I can do something with my life." From distant childhood dreams nursing sprang easily to mind.

With great care I perused the many courses on offer and selected the nursing assistant course as the most suitable one for me. So I pursued the qualification with firm resolve during evening classes over a period of two years. I was spurred on by bouncy enthusiasm carried on a wave of certainty that this was what I wanted to do.

I loved every minute, every inch of training. Indeed my life began to change inwardly, confidence replacing simplicity. When the exams burst upon me I passed with flying colours and slipped into my first post at the big hospital in Regina.

The Nursing Home where I'm at now is the biggest of its kind in the whole of North America. The place is vast with immaculate surroundings. We were a 700-bed institution but lately it has been cut down to 500 because the budget is apparently slightly up the creek.

The Home is not confined to geriatric inmates. A sad social norm prevails here in the North where working children discover that it's too much of a bind to have parents-in-need-of-care. The pursuit of careers became their major priority and they could not cope with Mom and Dad as well.

It's very different from the family situation back home where we Coloured and Black people lovingly care for our old folks. You cannot pound this kind of filial respect into the heads of Northerners.

As a consequence the Nursing Home takes people of all stripes – people who have been held in the highest social regard very often, and also people of not very considerable means.

In this kind of nursing you really need to watch every step you take because the patients can hit you and you have to know how to handle them. Mostly it's the ones who walk around flashing a dazzling smile your way one minute, then suddenly lurching out the next with blows to your solar plexus.

They don't know what they're doing and for you the shock is great because normally the person could be as quiet as a mouse in a hole. There are no warnings for us. Their minds can be lucid one moment and then suddenly change. Everything happens in a terrible flash.

The Head nurses have charts about the various conditions of the patients and treatments and these have a place in assisting us in our handling of them. Fortunately we are not required to do much for them because as Alzheimer sufferers they are able to do for themselves. Mind you, they might not want to stop piling clothes on while dressing themselves, but they would be mortally offended if we tried to assist them. In any case it is not part of our designated duty to do hands-on care for them.

The saddest thing for me about Alzheimer sufferers is that many of them were doctors, lawyers, professors and the like. They are only there because of being suddenly confronted by change they would sooner avoid but finally cannot escape.

I love to listen to some of the patients when they talk about their past lives. It is regrettable that we have such little spare time, but whenever an odd moment presents itself, I'd spend it listening to how they grew up, what their lives were like during the productive years.

There is always this need for someone to listen, to assist them in untangling their maze of words. Usually their recollection of detail is faultless. Admittedly not all the health care workers are good to them; perhaps that would be asking too much of human nature, but I have lots of patience and thoroughly enjoy sitting with them should time permit. In return I experience privileged glimpses into human hearts.

Our staff consists of registered nurses, assistant nurses and housekeepers. The latter clean the floors and put a shine to everything. Night duty begins with reports, just like in any hospital. After that we assistants start to load our night carts with fresh linen which we need lots of, for the patients with catheters, colostomies etc.

We then check each bed, looking after those with skin breakdown first. No person is excluded during these rounds. Each group of us is assigned 70-80 patients and a registered nurse is placed with each group. Though this is quite a large workload, we supply the needs of all. Medication is brought by the registered nurse who puts it down for us assistants to administer.

We have a round for bowel care and of course the colostomies have to be changed. Basic care at night makes nursing a very busy occupation. In addition we have paperwork to get through. I normally do mine around 3:30-4:30, because soon after that the place comes alive like an ant-heap.

The outstanding difficulty on night duty is the fact that while the majority of patients in your compliment are comfortably cocooned in their blankets, there are the ones who perpetually punch their call-light buttons. There is no way that these calls can be ignored because the only place for the light to be shut down is at the bedside.

When you hasten half a kilometre to get to the bed you find that it is merely someone lying there hollowed by loneliness, or wrestling with their own frailties, or crying and merely needing someone to hold their hand.

LAHLEKILE

Some of the patients are heart-broken because their people could not be bothered to come and see them, then when you happen to be the one to show a sliver of kindness, they pounce on you as though you are a life-saving straw.

PART 4 - ACHIEVEMENTS AND PROPOSALS FOR CHANGE

JANE

I remember back in England before I left to go to America, it was in an accident ward that we had an old patient there who was some sort of low-grade schizophrenic, very inadequate he was. He landed up with us because of some orthopaedic deformity. Now he'd been there for some weeks and then months without anyone being able to do anything about him. Meanwhile his vacuous melancholia sucked my heart dry.

I simply do not like loose ends. My resolve was to fix him up socially before I left the shores of Britain. This goal I pursued with promptness, verve and spirit. Firstly I phoned the Social Welfare, then psychiatry, then health clinics and so on, arguing my case with astute moderation.

The approach, I think, lies in ordinary action by ordinary people. That way you can alleviate human stress to effect change. Anyway I got him out and there's a subterranean satisfaction in knowing that I succeeded.

If I could change things it would be to teach people in health care how important the small things are. I know that today's student nurses have to devour many books and manuals and when they register they have lots of bars but they don't seem to see when a patient is upset or in pain. I'd really like to change this, to find something that approximates a solution.

Enmeshed in this is the importance of getting people to do things properly, like cleaning, which no one seems keen on anymore. To be fair I must say that I'm not sniping at junior nurses who have a lot to do, but nursing is astonishingly simple.

As an example, we had a maternity patient who had come in to be checked. She came in flat on her back and we were not sure what to do at first because all we had was very sketchy information from the referring hospital.

It was just on the lunch hour and I discovered that the patient was starving when I commenced to feed her. Along came someone who raved around me crying, "Now that is nursing!" Others came along to say things like "You're wonderful."

These remarks put me into a ferment. I was being praised to the rafters for basic nursing? I actually lay awake a few nights worrying about it. Is nursing not encumbered with cleaning, feeding, making the patient comfortable, and for this I had to be lavishly praised?

Another small illustration: Baby in a head box, drip up, analyser on, apnoea mattress in, infusion pump…all the wonders of modern science tra-la-la, and yet, filthy mouth. I cherish a sanguine hope that this will change.

You ask me for an overview of how I see nursing, having had my experience fanned out over three continents?

Well obviously if you go into the aspect of equipment then we in South Africa lag far behind the Northern

Countries. We all know that, how tightly squeezed we are in terms of money.

But making a comparison between private hospitals like St. Dominic's here, which I know because I worked there, then it falls far short of the sheer opulence of American hospitals. The furnishings and everything there is simply wonderful.

From an interpersonal point of view I'd passionately argue for the present holistic model of nursing as opposed to the hawkish military model with its cloistered traditions. Though I should hasten to add that there are good aspects in the latter, which we should mourn for.

However I'm a laid-back person who likes people. I'm really very easy-going and I find things are better now. We have crossed previously impenetrable boundaries from earlier times when nurses were given little choice.

Still, I think we need to know our hierarchy. Even if we are calling people by their Christian names we still need to give people the respect that's due to them. It is a root that goes down so deeply you can't pull it out.

I suppose the fact that we've got technology – all the modern machinery such as infusion pumps as opposed to the dreary old drips – that is a plus factor too. But I do think that out of the impetus of these developments came a lack of honest-to-goodness nursing. Patient comfort and well being remains the staple ingredient of nursing. That is something the older nurses knew how to achieve.

LAHLEKILE

PAMELA

It is difficult for me to pinpoint anything as an achievement really. One does what has to be done without giving it a second thought. It is only when seen through the eyes of other people that one's deed might be seen to be remarkable. Even today with the new concept of incident writing, the nurse is finding it hard to blow her own trumpet.

I once helped with the establishment of a local branch of Alcoholics Anonymous. It involved having to do home visits on a voluntary basis after hours, to support people who needed such a service. I also pioneered a pre-school centre for the Buffalo flats area. Such a need had become apparent when my eldest daughter stepped out of nappies.

I was the one who had marched briskly to the municipal authorities to request a plot of ground on which a prefab building could be erected. We had been promised such a facility by the Round Table.

A great many issues were slung back and forth for several dreary years until I slipped off the committee to channel my energies elsewhere. I know that you worked very hard (to the interviewer) for several years and actually got a day-care centre established but I am mentioning for the record that I had started it off.

EDITOR'S COMMENT

It took savage exertion to get the Tommorowland Day-Care Centre up and running. It was done with the assistance of the Rotary Club and a few dedicated members of the community. What rankles is that my efforts as an employee of the municipality at the time were completely overlooked by the shortsighted bureaucrats in charge of municipal affairs. Yet annually accolades are handed out to all and sundry.

PAMELA CONTINUES

If I had the power to change things it would be the 4-year course. The students ascend this academic mountain with such speed that you wonder how much of the material is mastered.

From my experience, we have to teach them so much. We had a sister who came to us who knew so little about the work despite orientation. One day it was required of her to do a survey of a squatter locale. All the sisters simply refused to come to her aid.

Their rationale was that she had all the knowledge of the 4-year course, how could *we* possibly be of use to her? Eventually someone from the office approached me and, willing horse that I am, I went along.

Purely from a basis of experience I had to take the lead, showing her how to take a head-count, how to list the adults separately from the children, the babies and the elderly. Then how to do an assessment of toilet facilities, employment, taps, animals etc. This is the type of information we gathered.

We found that all of them were unemployed, refuse was strewn all over and toilets were non-existent. Their main occupation was scavenging at the municipal tip. While water was begged, borrowed or stolen from neighbours with running water, children were constantly sent out to beg food from working people in the township, sharing their takings with the parents.

The highly qualified professional nurse was then able to compile a report from our findings, which hugely pleased the nursing service manager. Though her input had been zero all the credit went to her.

I would like to see the four-year course revised, to see them link the theory to the practical. I honestly believe that a serious re-think is necessary. Of what use is it to sport all the bars on your epaulettes and then you go into practice on shaky legs?

MERCY

Top of my list for change is attitudes.

Even with this integration, with the concept of a "new South Africa" it's all theory really. Where I am working now we have been fully integrated but the problem that sticks out like a sore thumb is who will be in charge? In the dark, dismal past (which was merely weeks ago at the time of this interview) there was always the situation of junior whites being placed in authority over senior blacks.

The new situation of integration has not been resolved at all.

The nursing service managers now say "You must all work together...." but this kind of lets-have-it-both-ways equivocation no longer impresses.

The attitudes have not changed. It is clearly the white nurses who are having problems. Issues of utter intractability now lie across their path.

Their need for rehabilitation cries out in the work situation. Here in the Out-Patient department when they see a white patient coming into the integrated climate three or four of them will flock in, in strutting style to determine how the white patient will be treated by the black staff members and they openly attempt to allay imagined patient-anxieties. I have not observed overt patient anxieties because of our black presence, which they see as an affliction apparently, but the nursing staff does.

I see them as thrashing about in the political undergrowth like trapped animals in the midst of a natural disaster such as floods. We black nurses are going to have to shake a few sacred apartheid cows if we do not want apartheid nursing to last into the next millennium.

I have not had any gender problems not having worked much with male nurses, only with doctors and there one could slip on a banana skin. Male doctors like to bark at nurses and get them into disarray but I've always operated on the belief that in practice we have to work well together. So far I've not experienced difficulties in this regard. There is undeniably the skin-colour problem of which they suffer a phobia but I find it easier to overcome this problem with doctors than with nurse administrators and their no-holds-barred emotionalism.

Things have got to change. We, belonging to the profession, are the instruments of change. If I had any power I would seek to change the mentality of nurses, turn it around from apolitical to ultra-political but outside party politics. Nurses must gain the perception that their problems are basically politically orchestrated.

I would love to be instrumental in changing the outlook of whoever is involved in the health situation. I could claw away the fog of rhetoric and broaden everyone's mind. Really I don't want to harangue, but nurses have been so indoctrinated that their vision begins and ends with whether the patient has had an intake and output and please to obey the rules! I find that abhorrent.

What they were not taught is that a nurse is a human being and as such she had got human rights. That is flat-out wrong. This wrong was perpetrated against all nurses and is being upheld seemingly into perpetuity. There is a glaring need to educate oppressed nurses in particular as to their human rights and what to do about the violation thereof.

In the not-too-distant past nurses were oppressed by nurses under the system of apartheid which favoured Whites. Yet it is *not* the oppressors of the past who are keeping nurses down now. The situation has eased somewhat since nurses are now recognised to be civil servants too.

The problem lies with nurses themselves who are unable to throw off the shackles of oppression. Nurses are scared. They remind me of the story of a monkey who was chained to a pole. The owner one day said, "There are so many monkeys running around I might as well free this one." So he freed his monkey who then ran around a few steps away only to return to the area of its imprisonment.

Like in Shakespeare's Julius Caesar, Cassius – when told that if Julius Caesar was going to be crowned he would become a tyrant who would torture him, the reply from Cassius was: "Cassius from bondage will deliver Caesar."

I say: "Nurses from bondage have got to deliver nurses."

MR T.

Gender problems abound in psychiatric nursing. Firstly, there is the distinction in labour. The male nurse is seen as the "muscle-man" who has to intervene with dangerous patients of either sex. Female care-givers tend to feel demeaned working in closed wards and they refuse to enter forensic wards saying, "We do not enter there, they will kill us...they will rape us..."

Secondly there is the resentment on the part of females toward male colleagues. The males are in the majority. They are able to argue points succinctly. Female colleagues rather give in easily to argument and sometimes swallow pride along with principles.

There seems to be an overwhelming fear that males in higher positions are going to marshal everything and disempower females in the process. The female attitude is often expressed along these lines. "They want to dictate things, this is not their field, why don't they go to the mines?" Such outrageous and repellent remarks commonly pop up in tearoom conversation.

Thirdly, upward mobility is controlled by the authorities that display a thin-skinned reaction to males with higher qualifications. The underlying reasoning seems to be: "He will be scorched by ambition. His quest for higher salaries and higher positions will be more imperative. We females should guard our territory..."

The fact that higher qualifications in nurses of both sexes are simply ignored, indicates that this is a threat to the white-on-top status quo. To be thus ignored is a bruising humiliation to nurses. In fact it is a blatant injustice, a notable flaw in apartheid nursing which will need to be corrected soon.

The 90's is a time that is both dynamic and unstoppable. My colleagues and I have nothing but good wishes for the progressive nurses of today, those who are opening the door to a new age in nursing. I wish them the very best.

MYMOENA

My heart leaps at your question concerning achievement because mine was a bonanza achievement as part of a group of four and we ought really to have our names flashed in neon lights had life been fair (gurgling laughter).

Well in community health nursing in those years, the curative services took precedence whereas to uplift the health status of the population we need the order of promotive-preventive-curative, like they had in communist China, but here we had it the other way around.

At one time four of us were chosen and given the unique responsibility of running the very first comprehensive health clinic at Heideveld on an experimental basis. If that was going to take off it would become the catalyst for further such services.

We became a new breed of innovators, reaching into dimensions of intelligence and understanding we never knew we possessed. Incredibly hard work was the driving force that propelled our success, for through team effort, Heideveld goes down in the medical history of our country as the first comprehensive health care delivery facility.

My colleagues were Lillian de Vries who headed the team, Jattiem, Moodley and I. What we had to do was to take the clinic out of the little compartments that City Health had rutted its services into – TB, Child Health, Dental and so on – we faced the daunting task of having to integrate all these under one roof and it was no picnic.

Our central preoccupation was to figure out how we could network ourselves and build up alliances, for we had to reconstruct the City Health's self-contained elements/units of health care delivery which had hived off into subcultures. Integration of services was the only plausible response to the new (global) demand for PHC.

To accomplish this task we had to display dynamism, which was not the core idea of nursing according to our training. So we had to shake off the vestiges of traditional South African nurse thinking. And we did it!

In the early 70's *we* gave birth to primary health care according to the concept sprouting from the historical Alma Ater conference. During those years even U.C.T. (University of Cape Town) did not have a chair for PHC and those doctors beat a pathway to *our* door to suss out from our grassroots experience the expertise needed to apply progressive principles in practise and so to forge a way forward for themselves.

Regrettably, as nurses, we did not have the skills at the time to document this vitally important experiment to add to the nursing knowledge base. Our raison d' etre was to act as welders in the practical arena. We were in the swim of things with more important fish to fry than writing up our deeds in books. So the doctors came to look at the situation with their fresh and detached eye and they were able to rake a rich harvest from our achievement.

To think about change somehow rubs me up the wrong way. If I had a chance to re-live my life I should not choose nursing because you cannot develop as a person within its narrow confines. I really blame the present iniquitous system for this. It forces us to become two people, to do one thing and to feel another: to say one thing and to think another. Now there is an all-out cry for democracy. Yet that word holds a meaning for oppressed nurses that it could not possibly have for privileged whites.

It is attitudes that must change first; there should be far more flexibility and openness. I believe that the young nurse must be given far more say. Space must be opened up for him and her to participate creatively in decision-making.

The female nurse especially, faces a more complex future if one looks at gender oppression as a factor she has to contend with too, on personal, social and professional levels. No matter how diverse females are as individuals, what we all have in common is our vulnerability as nurses and as women.

The modern nurse of both sexes needs psychological and political space to develop as we were prevented from doing, in order to gain deeper insights. If this is not done speedily, nurses may end up as a mediocre underclass.

AUDREY

I became interested in diabetes so I started attending conferences, arranging workshops for patient-education. It was not sufficient merely to provide tablets to patients who had no understanding of their treatment regime. Often they did not know why they had to come everyday. Eventually I came to be treated more as a consultant nurse when it came to diabetes.

If I could prioritise for change, remuneration would be top of the list. When I commenced training the shoe allowance was R6.00. Today in the 90's this allowance still stands at R6.00 despite the fact that the Rand has fallen out of bed. So I think that nurses' salaries must be increased according to their level of academic achievement. People who take time and money to study further should be rewarded.

The next thing is the gross shortage of nurses. Everybody is talking about the shortage but no one is doing anything about it.

They say "posts have been frozen" but the patients have not been frozen.

I always feel empathy with staff members whenever I work over weekends and I visit different wards. Take paeds for example. You'll find 55 babies with only two sisters, one assistant-nurse, and one staff-nurse. I believe that this gross shortage of manpower deserves attention at the highest level.

BILLY

My achievement lies in taking the extra mile for the patients whom I serve in the geriatric service. We organise outings for them on a quarterly basis. One such was a visit to the nursery where they were able to delight in plants, flowers and the craft shop. At another time we took them out for tea at the Marina Glen where the sunlight had lain as varnish on the esplanade.

For the 1993 outing the route was diverted to Fullers Bay on a golden November day. The sea had shone like silver paper under clear blue skies. At the very next clinic session they asked permission to have something said. Then I was told – to rapturous applause – how very much each and every one of them appreciated me. (The green eyes were suddenly moist with tears while her voice choked with emotion). They said, "My child, what you are doing for us not even our own children find the time to do." My heart swelled at what I recognised as the best, most wonderful compliment to me.

I've not had any gender problems as such although in my situation I work with two doctors who expect the geriatric clinic to run as smooth as an assembly belt but my patients are human and cannot be rushed. They see their nurse only once a month and bottle up the problems they'd like to discuss with her.

Change is urgently needed around hours, shifts, and salaries. I believe that nursing is not attractive enough for a modern era. Young girls today would not meekly accept the inadequate salaries. Why should they when the world has become their oyster?

I also do not agree with the 4D course, which is nothing more than a crash course as far as I'm concerned. They hop from TB today to geriatrics tomorrow, child health next and so on. In between they grapple with record keeping. I do not see how they can muster a cohesive train of thought, let alone seek underlying causes for the health problems they are confronting. The most glaring error in nurse training is to make them swot symptoms and carry out doctor's orders leaving their own judgement skills to lie fallow.

What lies very close to my heart when it comes to change is the operating arena. If a cosmic wand could empower me and make me nursing service manager of the Frere theatre system I should immediately set out to raze the present system to the ground, build it up soundly from the bottom and transform the atmosphere to one of healthy normality.

I'd wave my magic wand to annihilate the entire management structure including the doctors with their stifling attitudes. They never acknowledge our existence except with the frostiest of nods. They only see us in terms of pairs of hands that pass the instruments to them. On every other occasion they push us into the background unless forced to address us, then it is with razored elegance.

Not that we desire to be fresh with them, heaven forbid, but one needs to be recognised as a person. They'd have conversations with one another while taking everything out of your hands. I feel that doctors should recognise nurses more. We are not the nonentities that they try to make of us.

Nurses are unable to really grapple with this problem. We do large sections of specialised work – besides our nursing input – often filling in as doctors, social workers, physiotherapists or the like. Why are we not paid a just remuneration? Money is a very agreeable commodity providing you have enough over to splurge on mostly for basic needs and wants; it simply is not fair. The bottom line is that we are very specialised and should be paid on a par with doctors.

IRENE

As far as achievement is concerned, in my present capacity as nursing service manager I find that I've done well and have proved that as a black manager we are fully capable of being entrusted with such high-level responsibility and in maintaining standards and discipline required for a fully integrated hospital such as Settlers.

I think that whites, on the whole, believe that they are the only ones who can manage things. My immediate structure consists of four other white ladies. What I do every now and then is to draw on my black supervisors and bring them in on management meetings, to the corridor of power, at the same time to prepare them for the future. People these days want to see that their people are progressing.

Another problem is that when an issue arises the staff members do not feel free to raise it to a white person. So many times its been said to me, "You know, we feel we can come to you to discuss problems because you understand." So this could be another achievement perhaps, that I've established a line of communication in the hierarchy that flows up and down.

When it comes to change I would prioritise the conditions of service for nurses. In the past we were seen as domestics. We were not recognised as professionals and when you look at the salaries there has not been a significant change. Britain, for many years, has paid nurses for unsociable hours worked. Having been a theatre nurse myself I was out on call so many times without any extra pay. Weekends especially, you don't get any extra money for being on call, nor for public holidays.

The same applies to uniform allowance. We still get R6.00 for uniform and shoe allowance. As a nursing service manager I get R10.00 but recently I bought an outfit from Creative Fashions in Pretoria where I paid R850.00 for three skirts and two jackets, one with long, the other with short sleeves. I buy about three pairs of shoes a year and the R10.00 allowance does not take me anywhere.

LAHLEKILE

I am immensely concerned about the new curriculum. It's all very well for these girls to get the fantastic training but they get too much theory and not enough practical. If they come out, one minute they're a student, the next a sister. Previously you had to be a staff-nurse first and that was a good learning period for the novice though unfortunately it was abused somewhat due to nepotism. I really feel that the practical aspects of the curriculum ought to be re-evaluated. I remember that after an entire year of midwifery training I did not feel competent to be a midwife.

At Settlers' we have already experienced strike action 4 times running. In 1990, like a bolt out of the blue, the first strike occurred soon after Nelson Mandela was released from jail. The next one was called on 5 February 1991 then again on 3 and 4 August 1992 and again in June last year, the latter because of inadequate salary rise.

During this last strike I was lambasted on their posters, called a racist and told to step down. This was because I supposedly take on only so-called nurses.

Now although this action was a stinging slap in the face it failed to plunge me into mental turbulence. I have a selection panel and like in all walks of life you take the person with the best qualification for the job on hand. We consider symbols too because there are hundreds of matriculants walking around and a lot of these are unable to cope with nursing if they have not mastered English. This is not so much out of their own but because of the toll on their education as a result of Bantu Education, school boycotts and the social fragility of the townships.

Nevertheless, despite many of my black staff members having come on duty during the last two strikes, there were general assistants going around checking on this and intimidating the black nurses to leave. The potential damage of this action is so huge it is indescribable. During this time the white and coloured nurses were left alone.

The black nurses then made an extraordinary response. They did not allow the conflict to develop and reach unbelievable dimensions. What they did was to form a committee to which they called the shop steward, whom they then fired, having no mandate to speak for them. They wanted to confront NEHAWU on certain matters like their right to freedom of choice, their right to carry out their professional duties whereas the general assistants are not able to represent nurses on these matters

On the positive side I must say that though the strike catastrophes far exceeded anything foreseen by nurses, in Grahamstown there is the most fantastic support coming from the community at large. Church groups offer voluntary service. People phone in to ask, "Do you need any help?" That serves to bolster nursing morale. On the negative side the strikes have plunged the nursing profession into deep confusion, the sooner we are able to establish a new organisation representative of all the nurses, the sooner nurses will be able to weave a web of solidarity and protection for themselves.

RITA

One achievement I could happily document comes from the area of Primary Health Care, where I come from.

LAHLEKILE

For no apparent reason a decree was slapped on us to work on Saturdays. I regard this as grotesquely uncharitable since the individual does not belong to herself only but to a family and since the family is in fact a stable unit of society.

Prior to this the general assistants were found to owe hours, so they had to work these out on Saturdays. The norm was for all clinics to be closed over weekends. At our establishment the general assistants still worked a 40-hour week but it was split in such a way as to make them work on Saturdays. Professional nurses then had to take up duty to supervise the sweeping and cleaning of floors.

I deplored the prurience of the administrators, their slave-owner mentality. In fact I fell into a melancholy state of mind over this. I asked the workers and colleagues "Do you appreciate working like pack-horses without a break? Of course they did not. So I raised their awareness to the point where we could become proactive on the issue. A major change was effected.

Furthermore, another worthwhile cause for me to strive for was quality resources. I was active on the committees that enlightened the people as to the new concept of primary health care, giving them emotional amperage.

When I observed the nonchalance with which debris could be strewn around I realised that they needed to undergo a conversion. I then taught them that the hospital is a resource for the people and it would be in their best interest to take care of it.

So the heads of area committees and of street committees came together and began to process the clearing away of grime and debris. Our intervention altered their course. I enjoyed being involved in this progressive issue.

VALERIE

My first priority veers towards the cultural deficit in our educational programme. I still smart at the brazen manner in which peoples' rights were ignored with death and dying. I am especially hurt at the callous treatment of Hindu people when they lose a loved one, being a follower of this faith. I confronted nurses once as to what they were doing. "We're following typed notes" they replied but when I pressed them as to the source they did not know. "Have you consulted with Hindu people?" I asked. They did not, "We just thought this was the way it was done.

Hindu followers have rights when their loved ones die. These are:

♦ That the family be called and invited to perform last rites.
♦ That they may prepare the body using holy ash and the red dot both of which are important markings.
♦ That they be allowed to say prayers for the soul of the departed.
♦ That the deceased may be dressed in robes of the family's choice such as a wedding outfit, a christening robe, or any other clothes chosen by the family. They have the right to reject the cross on the

shroud as that is in conflict with Hindu symbolism. A holy person could be buried in traditional yellow robes.

I know that nurses have been laying out Hindu corpses without any respect for the traditions. This is nothing short of sacrilege.

I'm profoundly concerned too with the current nursing education system, which needs a total transformation. Our present system is not democratic, not as we enter 1998, the burning issues are not being addressed.

Most urgent of all is the problem facing the student nurses who had Bantu Education. They are grappling with adjusting and adapting to the nursing curriculum. South African nursing education needs to move swiftly into CBE (Community-based education). It needs as soon as yesterday, the introduction of problem-based learning programmes. I am profoundly concerned that we are still using old traditional evaluation' systems, which do not deal with the obnoxious Bantu Education shortcomings.

Take the language difficulty. Papers were set, without fail, in Afrikaans for Afrikaans speaking student nurses. Yet African student nurses are from Xhosa-based learning, so why are their papers not set in their language?

Bantu Education scrimped on mathematics and science. It pushed Agriculture, Bible Studies, Accountancy and the like. We should be providing academic support programmes to close the gap. These should focus on language acquisition and remedial education.

With regard to Human Rights violations, Nurses have never gone through a healing process. For me that's a great ethical problem. It is tremendously unsettling. Papers are being presented, books written by the score, but none are getting down to healing. We are negotiating, bargaining for more money and everything else but we are not effecting change in the nursing mindset. In nursing education we are doing the country a great injustice by not transforming. We should not be taking old problems into the new South Africa. We desperately need a new nursing education' dispensation.

I should like to bring out my own personal human rights deprivation suffered in the milieu of nursing education. As a lecturer I found myself exposed to builder debris during construction work at the institution where I practise. I had no history of asthma until directly exposed to dust, paint and whatever when the construction work began. My physiological reaction was extreme and raised the concern of my doctors who identified a problem of "exposure to an environmental hazard."

The official institutional response was adversarial. It was not accepted that my ill-health condition could be labelled as it had been, by two private doctors. Somehow that was taken as a reflection on the institution. The hospital doctor was informed of my case and without examining me she nevertheless recommended that I be redeployed to another college in another city.

They took a high-handed attitude rather than alleviate my situation either by stopping the construction until the doors closed for the December holiday or by allowing me sick leave where I could remain in a "safe and clean environment, " as was my right, until the hazard had passed.

I requested that the reports be forwarded to the Medical Superintendent who apparently responded in my favour (I was unofficially informed by a colleague manning our Sick Bay). Their "option" offered to me on a tray of bigotry had been rejected outright. I was not to be redeployed under any circumstances.

Yet the authority at the institution remained tight-tipped. Eventually I approached the principal to enquire as to the outcome. She responded that she was not aware that I needed a reply. When I confronted the institution's safety officer - who happened to be a member of my own community - she tried to pass the buck, saying she knew nothing of a safe environment as related to Human Rights. Her attitude indicated that she stood aloof from my problem. With a dollop of sarcasm I had to point out to her that it was possible to access the Occupational Safety Act to find out what peoples' rights were in this regard.

Yet another momentous concern is that of the bridging course. African student nurses doing this course are seriously disadvantaged, have mostly Standard V111 and are skimmed off small rural hospitals around the Province. We've put them into a mainstream education system. This is a horrific violation. What do we hope to achieve?

They are expected to do two years of the bridging course and then sail into the highly academic 4.D. I maintain that the issue of rural nurses was not addressed. In former years (before 1994) we had young staff nurses with Standard X. Classes then had 90% Standard X whereas today we have 20%. One of my current cadres of students is a male nurse of 57 years old with Standard V111.

The State approach is to upgrade staff nurses to registered nurse level. That will be the only route into the future, a comprehensive course for all practising nurses. (This excludes Nursing Assistants trained by hospitals. This training falls outside the gambit of nursing education).

The Council has a community nursing component in the future comprehensive 4D. They have allowed exit points. If the student exits for whatever reason at the end of the second-year level, she or he will be enrolled as a registered nurse. The bridging course will fall away.

My concern is that we have about 12000 staff nurses. We need to get them upgraded. They are probably the most disgruntled group in the nursing profession. We cannot blame them for going to the trade unions, which at least can speak out for them.

I really would like to raise community awareness about this problem. These staff nurses run the wards at night and act as registered nurses in many instances due to administrative problems such as staff shortages. They are good enough to do that in South African Hospitals. I have been a silent witness to their situation in the Province where I happen to be.

These staff nurses furthermore are being deprived of promotion if they happen to be of African ethnicity.

Whites and Coloureds are promoted to senior staff nurse level but here, in the urban setting not an African staff nurse. When I ask my students how many of them had been promoted, maybe one or two hands will be raised. That is pathetic. It indicates that the problem might be universal. Even in the Milk kitchen you will find senior staff nurses other than African. A travesty once again.

I should like to pose this question to South Africa at large. What is to become of this cadre of service providers? Is their situation of terminal enslavement acceptable in the democratic South Africa?

Hierarchical Oppression

STATURY BODIES: The South African Nursing Council (SANC), the licensing Body, was as far removed from nurses as the anthropological perception of GOD was to primitive people. [The reader is referred to the story of Ella]. SANC was seen and heard only when individuals erred legally and required punishment or official reprimand. Court proceedings were set up in a circus-like atmosphere whenever nurses had to be tried by SANC. Colleagues from near and far were encouraged to attend these proceedings probably as sombre warnings to themselves not to cross the statuary rules and regulations in any way.

Nursing was governed by double standards. For example, at Frere Hospital in the Eastern Cape the midwifery students for many years were not allowed to cross the threshold of the white theatre if they happened to be darker pigmentation. Scores passed the midwifery exams without the theatre experience yet SANC did nothing about that blatant deprivation.

Matrons [currently designated as nursing service managers]

Editorial comment:
What has been revealed about matrons is the painful truth as experienced by the oppressed nurses of South Africa. However, there were exceptions.

I should like to record that before my retirement from the profession in the late 1980s, my late husband's illness had become terminal. I was in Cape Town at the time, gaining experience in Adolescent Services. I had to hastily return home, but found my passage blocked at the regional CPA office in Port Elizabeth.

Subsequent to my secondment to the new Administration in 1994 I speedily discovered who had refused to give me a post then, despite my experience, tertiary education and excellent record in community health nursing [PHC], none other than a white nurse at the helm of administration then.

Meanwhile, the Cape Town admin people began to pull strings on my behalf. Frere Hospital was contacted. The matron of that time was a Ms Van der Merwe, who was greatly revered by nurses. She immediately opened a post for me, proclaiming that I was "a Frere girl" and deserving of assistance.

After my secondment to the new administration a while later, The Frere matrons heard about my husband's suffering and contacted me telephonically to ask if I required any assistance. As a consequence they provided me with the service of a secretary who remained with me until my retirement.

I'd like to emphasise that these matrons have earned my enduring appreciation for the magnificent support they gave me at a time when I was most vulnerable. Though the general nursing experience of matrons was far from pleasant, I wish to record that there were two sides to the same coin.

The history of matrons is studded with anomalies. Gross abuse of power can be laid at the door of these power-figures – they could be inaccessible, unapproachable, unfriendly and solemnly exercising the creed of their generation which was naked racism.

Racist attitudes in nursing were transported to the African continent by European missionary nurses (with exceptions in rare cases) and through a process of acculturation, infused into the collective breast of South African matrons (again with rare exceptions) who became predominantly white Afrikaner women.

A marked cruelty that they inflicted on this generation of young people, as they did on the previous one, was to underfeed them. Nurses from the best of homes had to endure meals that were scanty and dull.

Another mode of oppression was to close the door of nursing with dreadful deliberation after training. Hence black nurses had the greatest difficulty in securing posts. Similarly these matrons displayed an unbound capacity (and still do) to refuse nurses the opportunity to study further while in posts. They would firmly put down anyone who stood up for their rights. It was doubly deplorable that no freedom of expression was tolerated.

Matrons of this period were notoriously reluctant to espouse new protocols. Signs of obsolescence showed in hospitals where they continued to use old dressing packs deep into the SOS along with sporting old unenlightened attitudes.

It has been revealed through the interviews that promotion was granted to blacks that were conservative and willing to perpetuate the status quo. Black-on-black oppression is a new reality that has awesome implications for the future.

Together, the matrons of this period had a retrogressive effect on nursing and can be labeled as having been politically warped. They are directly responsible for the crosscurrents that prevail in every work situation where black and white are required to rub shoulders. They are responsible - as role models - for the black-on-black oppression of the late 90s.

Nepotism ground down with relentless force. This anomaly was most evident in salary discrimination. The first protest ever raised at Groote Schuur hospital in the early 70s was as a direct result of a salary increase for white nurses only. The relentless persecution, which the SANC was able to exercise against the nurse who led the strike, will blot the copybook of South African nursing in perpetuity. [The reader is referred to the story of Enid]. Fortunately the victim had clung with grim determination to the last shreds of dignity and had survived, be it in another country.

LAHLEKILE

Affirmative Action

The extreme complication for contemporary nurses is the fact that the middle-management [the floor matrons] are said to be blocking applications for promotion against the stated intention of the African National Congress that affirmative action is for all those who are not white. These floor matrons have made affirmative action a loaded phrase in nursing, espousing the cause that it is meant for African nurses only, leaving the other categories sorely provoked. This represents an old threat in new clothes. It seems feasible that the criteria of skilled management and fair play could be tossed through the window, with this political distortion.

Difficulties In Psychiatric Nursing

Lack of upward movement poses a difficulty in that the progressive individual becomes limited in the ability to develop subordinate staff.

Colleagues are often resistant to change. Here a major priority should be to bring understanding and insight to a patient rather than to create a dependency by doing things for the patient. Such dependency is unsustainable from a nursing point of view since the patient has to be returned to the family and the community as a functional being.

Control and management of a department - such as the hygiene of wards for example - is often allowed to supersede patient needs. Non-nursing departments can further cause setbacks to patient recovery. The case was raised of Stores causing lengthy setbacks when new equipment such as steel beds were ordered. The employees there did not easily believe that the mentally ill were deserving of better resources.

Domination by people "with tunnel vision" loomed as a difficulty. In the early 60s a nurse could not sit down to read a newspaper to a patient in the hope of getting him or her to react to life. Supervisors were all too ready to pounce on such a nurse, saying that they should not snatch at relaxation while on duty. That attitude has changed somewhat.

Resistance to develop in terms of updating of knowledge can be problematic. Quality care seems not to be universally cherished as an ideal. One interviewee decided to leave "the skeleton of psychiatric nursing" in the proverbial cupboard and concentrate on development instead.

Gender Problems

There were no problem in this regard between nurses, only between nurses and doctors who were mostly white males. In psychiatric nursing though, gender problems were more clearly defined. There is a distinction in labour. Male nurses are regarded as "muscle-men" who have to intervene with dangerous patients of either sex. Female colleagues show resentment towards their male colleagues in this field since males are in the majority by far. Apparently the fear is that males will gain superiority over females and would disempower them from a higher vantage point.

Training

Curriculum Characteristics: Examinations were PTS, PRELIM, INTERMEDIATE and FINAL. Prelim was withdrawn, apparently after protests forwarded by letter to Pretoria, that Blacks were deliberately failed to keep the numbers down. Nurses in Umtata were assisted by young lawyers of the day to write the letters to SANC. [Cape Town respondent, unfortunately my case-notes were lost]

Nursing etiquette received the highest priority, with great stress laid on respect for elders and for senior nurses. Similarly the caring aspect of nursing was prioritised. Socialisation of nurses aimed at inculcating the quality of humility. It is not inconceivable that this was to ensure the subjugation of nursing to the medical mode of health care delivery. The goal was achieved since nursing was dominated by religious compulsion (throughout the century) expressed through Christianity.

In general the standard of training was perceived to be good. It allowed space for further growth and development. Training eroded latent suspicion, which may have hung over from earlier unenlightened times. It brought the realisation that western medicine "can do wonders for people" as one interviewee put it.

Problems In Training

Apartheid was rife in the 60s and continued throughout the two decades under discussion. All tutor posts were held by whites. Just as in practice a junior white could give instructions to senior nurses, so too was white superiority entrenched in nursing education. Black sisters in colleges were designed as "sister-tutors." One interviewee remembers with excitement when the first black nurse educator arrived on the scene at Livingstone Hospital.

The sister-tutors are remembered fondly for having had nurturing attitudes towards their students. They provided the emotional support so lacking in nursing education up to that point in time. An interviewee related how they suffered under an Afrikaner tutor at Conradie Hospital and how delighted they had been when she eventually departed for a life in farming, giving them a respite from her tempers.

THE LAST FORTY YEARS

TRENDS FOR THE PERIOD

The reader is reminded that the nursing struggle has been documented and is amplified by nursing testimonies in this chapter. The difficulties were simply mind-boggling. For greater clarity, these difficulties are grouped under headings. They must be seen to reflect on the broad experience of the South African oppressed nurses even though in some instances white nurses suffered to some extent. The military mode of training as well as the medical mode of health care delivery, affected all nurses irrespective of race.

Nursing Hours

The unsociable hours - especially weekend duty - imposed severe restrictions on social life. Young people had to sacrifice their sport programmes, social clubs and the like, without any compensation such as provided in Britain.

Remuneration

Remuneration was one of the biggest bones of contention, which remains unaddressed at the close of the period. Discrimination between doctors' and nurses' salaries can be seen as the cause of the alienation between these categories of health care providers. Furthermore the salary differentials on the basis of race caused disharmony and bred racial hatred amongst black nurses towards their privileged counterparts.

Racial Oppression

To nursing administration the implementation of "white superiority" was a value as fundamental as the world is round. Racial oppression took on many forms in the various work situations, as told by the nurses of the period.

Priorities For Change

In view of the immense difficulties experienced by this generation of nurses one could be forgiven for appealing to all the stakeholders in health care - whether as providers or as consumers - that their suggestions be treated with the seriousness that it deserves.

- Change the mental outlook of nurses from "a-political" themselves, to "ultra-political" to enable them to challenge the system collectively.
- Change the outlook of health planners generally. Nurses feel obscurely cheated when they are not

consulted as a professional body. Though SANA's demise is imminent, a Transitional Nursing Committee does exist, representing all the nurses of the country, including the former homelands nurses. This body should be approached during the transitional period of reconstruction. Psychological and political space needs to be opened up for nurses.

- The single, most important determinant of status and rights in South African nursing has always been race. Eliminate racism not only from the statute book but in practice too. Include ethnic discrimination in practice.

- Give aspiring nurse-managers a trial period. Time will then reveal their suitability or not, for higher positions.

- Change the leadership - cleanse the enmity. Nurse managers need experience; they are largely accustomed to manage townships. Managers should be able to relate to colleagues, subordinates, patients, students and the community. They should display a willingness to pilot new protocols.

REMUNERATION is a crucial issue in terms of

- Non-discriminatory salaries in terms of race.
- Rewarding people according to qualifications.
- Upgrading nursing salaries realistically.
- Bringing shoe and uniform allowances in line with market realities.
- Stopping the economic exploitation of the nurse under the cloak of "professionalism."
- Eliminating salary discrimination between doctors and nurses with differentiation only where surgical procedures are concerned.

Curriculum Review In Terms Of

- Traditional socialisation unacceptable for the new South Africa.
- Meaningful participation of nurses required.
- Practical aspects to be re-evaluated.
- Psychiatry to be taken out of the 4D course.
- Modernise the educational structure and unshackle it from Pretoria (the statutory structure).
- Ensure that upward mobility occurs along specialised lines and not merely in administration.
- Change the statutory bodies; change the nursing Act.
- Important to have an organisation that stands for nurses.
- Study patient-needs. Quality care is not possible without resources.
- Public attitudes to be changed. Para-professionals who are accepted by doctors are seen as glamorous figures while nurses who are bossed and bullied by doctors have come to be regarded as a kind of underclass worker. Unless young nurses are shaped up as professionals in their own right they will by-pass the door of nursing, causing the intake to plummet. No doubt with disastrous results.
- Allow sabbaticals. Expose young people to nursing in other countries during an internship.

CHAPTER 4 - SOUTH AFRICAN NURSING IN TRANSITION

PART 1 - ANCEDOTAL ACCOUNT

FROM APARTHEID TO DEMOCRACY

Transition arrived on the nursing doorstep as a process which none of us understood very clearly. Soon after the magic day of President Mandela's inauguration, the print and electronic media erupted with hype about the new political elite imploding on the social scene.

Johannesburg and surrounding areas acquired a new name, which had a gutteral flavour as though plucked from a German lexicon. "Gauteng" suddenly boasted a "first lady" in the person of the premier's wife, Judy Sexwale.

An Eastern Cape newspaper screamed: "BAUTY GOES BAREFOOT" when a female politician appeared in the Legislative Assembly wearing traditional Xhosa clothes, lots of beads, no shoes, and a new surname – *Balindlela.* I was naturally ecstatic, having been friends with her in the pre-democratic era. Somehow, under the political regime of the Ciskei, she had decided to relocate to the Transkei those years and I lost track of her.

Television brought the visual of an "imbonge" stamping his feet in tribal ceremony. Never before had a praise-singer been allowed in the hallowed portals of the South African Parliament. It was a visual that probably jolted John Soap and his wife out of their political coma.

LAHLEKILE

In the narrow world of the hospital arena, where black and white occupied different worlds within the same space, the "them versus us" syndrome took on new depths of depravity.

We wanted to express the tumultuous excitement surging within us while *they* behaved as though some fearful calamity had befallen them.

When the jungle drum [hospital grapevine] conveyed the news that the new Minister of Health was to be a black female, our cup truly ran over, while 'they' retreated into sultry sullenness or aggressive predictions of gloom. "Where can I find more soap?" asked a general assistant of her white supervisor. "Ask Mandela" was the sour reply.

In an extreme case, a clinic sister refused to take the public holiday granted to state employees, preferring to come to work in a place normally closed on public holidays. She spent the time standing on chairs revamping curtains. When weeks merged into months, it became increasingly clear that our newfound happiness was as short lived as a roller coaster ride.

Editor's Note:

In April of 1994 I was swiftly seconded out of my post at Frere Hospital and appended to the new Health Administration in Bisho. Quite unexpectedly I found myself in the company of progressive doctors, mostly from exile.

I was given an office in East London, a car and virtual freedom from routine: The situation provoked a mixture of admiration and envy amongst colleagues who soon dubbed me "the one who flew over the cuckoo's nest."

My initial brief from the new Minister of Health's office was to join other provincial representatives in promoting a campaign entitled *TOWARDS A CARING HEALTH SERVICE*. Later I became the provincial coordinator for Health Promotion.

I am able to provide merely an anecdotal narrative of transition from apartheid to democracy. Other observers would have different perspectives. In my imagination, as I write, I sit like a naughty gnome on a rope ladder stretching down from the sky, observing the unfolding events as South Africans crossed minefields, or so it appeared.

Suddenly, new socio-political actors became visible. Our daily vocabularies had to take in all the buzz words: *accountability,* *transparency,* *participative democracy*...Disabled people were referred to by some *as physically challenged*...short people as *vertically challenged* and blind people as *visually challenged*. There was sufficient material to keep stand-up comedians in lucrative jobs for months.

In the nursing world, 'Homeland' colleagues suddenly appeared from behind the "iron curtain" of apartheid, some straight into positions of authority. At a subsequent national conference, a nurse described their situation with the terse comment, 'We were all trained in South Africa and then thrown into the bushes!'

Very soon, nurses came to realise that a career ladder was in place. There it stood, enticingly so, before the mind's-eye of every deprived nurse in the land. Everyone wanted to savour what it felt like to earn a decent salary, moreover "to be on top." Affirmative action became the hot potato that would reverse the swing of the pendulum, so we were told.

Before the election there were approximately 180,000 nurses in the Republic of South Africa of which 78,000 were registered nurses and midwives. These officers now found themselves flanked by thousands of colleagues formerly invisible.

Suddenly the race was on, the entire pack jostling to get up the ladder by fair means or foul. Bitter dog - eat - dog scenarios began to unfold in the workplace. Those secretly frothing with jealousy began to tunnel holes for others to fall into. I was in line for such onslaught but refused to become a victim. It was like a virus entering a computer. There was a real potential for the conflicts to create bureaucratic turbulence, which could lead to professional suicide. In fact this was soon to happen in the former Transkei.

The first phase of the process was characterised by endless meetings, committees, commissions, *strikes!* In our province, Bisho - home of the new administration - became the attractive flower for swarming hives of bees from the five capitals - Port Elizabeth, East London, Queenstown, Umtata, Kokstad.

The term "firefighting" arose from the ranks of those in authority. They were firefighting with all their might when strikes broke out in the old Ciskei early in 1995. Democracy was a ravenous tiger out on the prowl. Old grievances had festered into ripe boils. Pus was flowing.

Then the new Parliamentary salary scales were disclosed. This was extreme provocation to the "starving masses" of the revolution. Dialogue about the "gravy train" reverberated from taxis to shebeens, from coffee rooms to boardrooms and bars. Everyone craved a slice of the pie, no less the nursing fraternity who always felt themselves to be economically exploited. The *gravy train* debacle acted as a detonator to their resentment.

Though I was an extremely small cog in the wheel, I had high visibility in various parts of the province, being engaged in dialogue with the public. I presented for discourse the new three - tiered structure of a unified health system.

I soon discovered that the buzzwords meant little to people outside the department. Expectations had been raised by the landslide victory of the African National Congress, and people were chaffing over the slow delivery of promises put out by the Reconstruction and Development (RDP) manifesto.

The disadvantaged – the 'poorest of the poor' were expecting houses, water and electricity and why was this not happening? I found myself serendipitously in the frontlines as it were, so that the year 1995 became the most challenging, yet exhilarating year of my entire career.

I'd like to briefly describe a health related intervention that my office was called upon to make. The office had developed from the single task of coordinating for the campaign 'Toward a Caring Health Service' to one with a complex public relations character.

LAHLEKILE

I was advised by a coterie of colleagues from environmental health, occupational health, and administration staff. Everyone assisted, so that one felt cosseted by the strong support-base in East London. Individuals representing community organisations began drifting in to talk about a "way forward" for their particular concerns.

One day the management committee of a hospital in the former Transkei called upon me to attend a meeting without stipulating an agenda. Apparently I was called out of sheer desperation when all else had failed. I was not exactly brimming with enthusiasm for I suspected that I had to listen to a grievance, something not actually within my mandate. However upon consultation I was told. "When the people call we need to respond, if only to listen to what they have to say."

Nothing prepared me for what lay ahead. I was truly aghast when the burden of a hospital in crisis was flayed open. Other than the night nurses none of the staff were working the night shifts. The stoppage had occurred when homeland barriers had clashed with the political liberation. Health workers had then learned that their counterparts in the Republic of South Africa were receiving special allowances for night duty. They demanded that the matter be instantly redressed.

Without night duty staff there was no security at the hospital, no clerks to do the administration, no fireman and so on. Without a fireman there was no steam in the pipes, consequently no hot beverages for patients but far worse, no operating theatre facility. Patients coming in severely injured in accidents simply died for lack of surgical intervention.

If you died during the night your body might be passed into the care of private morticians. Since the hospital mortuary served its own and four other towns, six mortuary shelves were wholly inadequate.

When your folks arrived next day to see you, they would suffer not only the shock news that you had slipped off your mortal coil, but that your body had been placed elsewhere and no one quite knew where, because the hospital had not a scrap of stationery to have written down the details, nor the staff or the time. The relatives would then travel the rural surrounds in public transport and often return to the hospital around 5pm to state wearily that they had not located the whereabouts of your remains.

Once the hospital grievance had been tabled I was taken on ward rounds. First we stopped at the laundry where disconsolate workers were grappling with the task of hand washing piles of tattered linen. After seeing several broken down machines I was led outside to witness a mountain of new blankets rotting in the sun. Those could neither be done by hand nor could it be left inside to be a health hazard to the workers.

In the ground floor wards the shock hit my spine like a physical blow. It might have been less traumatic had one suddenly been plunged neck deep in ice. As the scenes played themselves out before my eyes it was like viewing the horrors in Schindler's List. The difference was, that you could then use the remote to turn it off. When the hospital administrator witnessed my tears running unchecked, he called a halt to the tour saying, "If you've seen one ward you've seen it all."

It was unforgivable that I could have lost control in the eye of the public, but of the all pressing concerns none had gripped me so profoundly as the sight of whimpering babies, lying mostly naked in drab little cots in unheated rooms.

Grievous as the situation of that hospital was, it merely echoed the scenario in rural hospitals elsewhere in the former 'homelands'. Administration worked itself bleary eyed to redress the massive obstacles in the way of patient comfort but this was against the backdrop of a 7½ million (Rand) deficit in the health budget of that homeland.

Due to my intervention, a delegation from the Butterworth Hospital was seen by an officer who was acting in the capacity of Deputy Director of Health Services. Protocol required that they took the grievances to the recently appointed Regional directors but they were seen at provincial level at my request.

We learned then that the potential damage of any strike action is so vast as to be almost incalculable. The problem was in fact far bigger than the province could handle itself. Officers with the highest designations had been to that hospital and much was being done, but it could not be set right overnight.

One happy outcome of the intervention was that a few micro changes were effected such as the replacement of laundry machines after architects and other planners were sent in. There was a misperception - which amused me very much - that it was my intervention that had brought about the changes. I was hailed as the "Patricia de Lille"* of the Transkei. Whereas in fact it had been an all-out effort from the very highest level of the Department.

[*Patricia de Lille was a parliamentarian with explicit views].

In 1995 new salary increases for health care providers was disclosed. All hell broke loose. The 5% was viewed as an insult in the face of the gravy train debacle. Strike action erupted in Gauteng and spread alarmingly. Firefighting became the major priority for administration from national to provincial levels as far as the former Transkei, where all health workers were unceremoniously called out.

It was not a call that could be ignored except at extreme personal risk. Not after what had been done to nurses during the 1992 strike in the former Transvaal. [Incidentally, that was a case recounted to me by journalist Musa Zondi, who said with great feeling: "they were burned to ashes"].

Communication between the militant union nurses and the state broke down in the face of a verbal slap from President Nelson Mandela. Nursing was treated like a recalcitrant female child who needed a fatherly scolding. I see the presidential attitude of that time as an outgrowth of the social system, the "I versus you" pattern of dealing with conflict, the pattern unwittingly tinged by gender and cultural overtones.

Similarly the Minister of Health, in user-friendly style, tried but failed to achieve a plausible intervention amid the adversarial atmosphere. Her efforts were rewarded by uncomplimentary placards appearing on television news programmes for all the country's nurses to buy into.

Primetime debates were conducted in which impartial TV journalists engaged major stakeholders from state and civil society in seeking solutions. I gained the impression that many of the participants perceived the nursing struggle as a purely professional malaise. It was an attitude that reinforced customs and values no longer acceptable in a democratic milieu.

As the weeks went by and the hospital death statistics rose, the Eastern Cape Department of Health and Welfare seemed to have reached the end of its tether. A salvo was fired directly to the striking nurses: Unless they returned to duty by a clearly specified date they would be considered to have dismissed themselves.

This directive naturally caused an agonising flutter. Some nurses risked life and limb to return to duty wearing mufti as a measure of protection. The bulk remained out on strike, admitting long after the event in a press statement, that they had been 'cynically manipulated by activists with political agendas'. Sheer, unadulterated pessimism ensured continued resistance. In the final analysis 6000 nurses had virtually dismissed themselves, losing valuable pension benefits in the process.

Meanwhile to the rest of the country's nurses, the Minister of Health came out with pledges of reform.

Since hope springs eternal in the human breast, most of us probably chose to believe that constitutional change was the surest path to social change. It was not very difficult for those in normal circumstances to continue with the pattern of conformity until April 1996. It would then be clear which way the cookie would crumble.

Within the nursing profession it should be an urgent concern of DENOSA, the new Nursing Association that replaced SANA, to use its leverage to promote the 'substantive equality for all' as promised in the Constitution. This can be done if the political will is there to have every person in the health care delivery system, at whatever level, oriented fully to the human rights framework, with gender-equality training included.

LAHLEKILE

PART TWO - FROM APARTHEID TO DEMOCRACY

FROM SANA TO DENOSA

Editor's Note:

Transition was effected after three national conferences. It should be noted that several organisations had mushroomed outside the traditional SANA, CINA and TRANA [SA, CISKEI and Transkei nursing associations]

In the Eastern Cape, which historically was the bedrock of nursing education for black women, there arose the organisation called the Democratic Association of South African Nurses [DASAN]. DASAN was ably chaired by Mr Tyalimpi of Queenstown, and carried the progressive view. During the last year running up to the first transitional conference, the chairman was Mr Dan Masala. For some time I was its secretary. Ms Dorothy Matabeni who serves on DENOSA, was one of the founder activists of DASAN.

As active members of DASAN, we were exceedingly proud of its constitution, drawn under the able hand of Advocate Louise Swanepoel. A copy of DASAN's constitution was handed to the incoming transitional committee. That constitution paved the way for the evolution of a progressive nursing association.

In February 1992 more than 20 nursing organisations were brought together in the first national consultative conference representative of the nurses-in-struggle. This initiative was taken by the Durban branch of the

CONCERNED NURSES OF SOUTH AFRICA (CONSA) who had secured funding for this event from the Kellogg's Foundation.

Nurses came from various parts of Africa and Europe to throw a lifeline to their colleagues-in-struggle. Most notably Dr Kupe, from the University of Botswana, came along as a representative of the ICN [International Council of Nurses].

The conference was opened under the eye of television cameras by two foremost nurses of our time, Mrs Albertina Sisulu, who delivered the keynote address, and Miss Glenda Weldschutte of the Western Cape, who chaired the opening. [Glenda was the only nurse who'd been selected to serve on the Truth and Reconciliation Committee].

Throughout most of the conference the atmosphere was pregnant with venom and hostility. South African nurses were worlds apart, divided by racism, ethnicity, xenophobia, language and politics! Also playing a prominent supportive role were scores of other activists, including doctors and union representatives.

The task of chairing across two days proved to be extremely challenging for the chosen team as the organisers had probably suspected. SANA was vociferously identified from the beginning as *'public enemy number one.'* Whoever chaired, got caught up in the dichotomy of traditional loyalty to SANA, and the need for fraternal relations with CONSA and the rest of the audience.

LAHLEKILE

Pro and anti SANA factions were equally belligerent. It was in the main an audience baying for blood, SANA's blood. Notes of angry protest began to rain down on the conference table before the first day ended. Acerbic questions peppered the agenda.

Fortunately the chair rotated frequently enough to provide relief to chairpersons who were under relentless pressure. Someone on stage [from TRANA] attempted to deflect the anger by introducing religious songs, but nurses refused to be enticed into mindless response. Dr Kupe was able to hold audience attention and did much to forge peace.

At one time Albertina Sisulu leaped on to the stage to curb a ragged outburst of shouting. "Comrades" she began, with perfect calm and equanimity. No one heeded her call as noisy rhetoric flew back and forth among the factions. "Comrades!" This time she raised her voice peremptorily yet was unable to gain the ear of the audience. At that time a howl of rage went up from a faction seated near the front. Southern Transvaal was verbally stoning SANA, demanding that its delegates be made to leave the hall.

"Comrades!" thundered Albertina Sisulu above the hubbub. Her voice carried a tone that brought the tumult into a sudden surprising silence. Then came the most amazingly meek, multitudinous response. "Mama?" cried the crowd, suddenly knee-capped into a child-like stance by the cultural inflection of motherly tones.

In firm voice she asked provocatively, "Did you not say that you want SANA to be accountable to this conference for the grievances you wish to air? Variously dazed, the subdued audience responded affirmatively allowing itself to be led like a child by its mother.

"Did you not write letters to the table demanding that SANA should speak?" Mrs Sisulu asked with dogged persistence. Again she had an affirmative response. "Now you want SANA to leave? Is that democracy? Comrades I request a mandate from you please. You will be democratic and allow SANA its democratic right to speak or we turn our backs on democracy and close the conference. What shall it be? I require your mandate now."

The mandate was an item most hotly debated in arguments slung back and forth across the hall between pro and anti-SANA factions. In the final analysis the majority opted for the democratic approach saving a terribly messy situation.

By that time nursing professors had been brought in to assist the delegates who had faced the angry crowd and been brought close to choking point by hostile audience reaction. It was not surprising to learn a few months later that Dr Bruwer, the head of SANA at the time, had resigned shortly after the conference "for health reasons."

Meanwhile, Dr Kupe spoke as a representative of the ICN. She made it clear that South Africa would not be accepted back into the international fold either as a white or black organisation, but as a body of unity comprising both races and all ethnicities.

Many riveting papers were presented. In addition, the Congress of South African Trade Unions [COSATU] brought the prospect of three possible options to nursing awareness. These were: *To democratise SANA; To join existing trade unions; To form a separate structure for nurses.*

By the time the third national conference took place, nurses had opted to form a separate structure resting on two legs, a union and an association leg. Meanwhile nurses from the USA had spelled out that the two-legged approach was currently a popular mode for overseas nursing organisations. They also raised awareness of nursing unity through a slogan, 'NURSES UNITED WILL NEVER BE DEFEATED.'

Consa delegates standing at the back of the hall took this up in a thumping bellow. For an appreciable length of time most of the audience joined in. That was stimulating. The demolition phase was in progress and we were virtually dancing around the ashes. Heart-stopping stuff!

Part 3 - Structural Oppression

The following information below is a product of the first conference workshop.

Control of Knowledge by Race and Class

Ethics and professionalism was based on the Florence Nightingale era. During the Crimean War, traditional cultural attitudes influenced the nursing profession to the extent that British nurses as women, had to scrub walls and floors and perform all the other domestic tasks traditionally accorded to women and girls. Florence Nightingale's 'Notes on Nursing' – a first in the world – reinforced this ethic that was later transported to South African shores by the missionary movement.

Few authentic black role models, if any, appeared in South African nursing literature. Nurses were trained on the premise that Henrietta Stockdale was the country's most venerable role model.

The idea was tabled at the first national conference, after a workshop, that history evolves slowly, is written from an individual perspective and is presented with a particular class and race bias.

Editorial Note:

I concur with the above contention.

In the run-up to the first democratic election, I was approached by the editor of a CINA nursing newspaper to produce for its consumers, articles relevant to nursing.

LAHLEKILE

After a while I was offered a column that I entitled *'FLIP SIDE UP'*

In this column I addressed issues such as the enforced membership of SANA. It was an issue that activist nurses were tackling at every given opportunity. In the former Republic of South Africa membership of Sana was made mandatory to getting an appointment processed.

The editor of 'The Light', as the newspaper was named, was approached by a SANA representative, who attempted to put a spoke in the wheel. However, she was invited to treat the newspaper as any other, by writing to him [Mr Sydney Mafa] as editor to voice their complaints. He warned though, that he would give his columnist the space to respond. Interesting to note is, that no one in fact took up the offer.

When the Nursing Act was eventually amended, compulsory membership was dropped, a decided victory for nursing activism in South Africa.

During this time, I was indirectly courted by one of the more friendly nursing academics, Professor Ilana Uys. She had put forward a suggestion to the SANA rep of our region, that I be persuaded to write for their Nursing News. It was a suggestion that could not raise a spark of interest in me.

The crux of the matter is that I too would have written from a particular class and racial bias. This is what the nurses were highlighting with regard to historical literature.

The Socialisation Process

The fact that nurses are together all the time was seen as 'contrived' by the conference participants. Not only are nursing students bunched together in classrooms and hospitals, but in Nurse's Homes as well. Socialisation imbues nurses with a value system as the system defines an ideal nurse. 'We are challenging that ideal' said the rapporteur during the plenary.

Ageism is entrenched in the socialisation process. There is the notion that those who are older have greater authority, whereas if you are young you are assumed to be impulsive and not to be trusted.

Nurses learn quickly that they are not rewarded if they challenge the system. Literature was geared towards religious values based on Christianity. Furthermore, an 'a-political stance' was fed into the nursing psyche from day one.

The Bureaucratic System

The hierarchy was described as a 'pyramid' with white males at the top and all nurses below. The medical model of health care delivery was doctor-dominated. Nurses carry out 'doctor's orders' rather than participate in seeking solutions for ill-health conditions. Yet the UNISA curriculum took aspiring graduate students through twelve courses at great financial sacrifice, not to mention the time-consuming academic burden. Still, they were not permitted to practice after getting their degrees, other than in the handmaiden role. Matrons give orders from above despite the fact that they too, fell under the domination of the male. To be noted is that the bureaucracy invariably favours whites.

Legislation

The two statutory bodies, SANA and SANC, were structured forms of oppression. You had to belong by law. It was a means of entrenching white supremacy. At first, only whites were allowed to serve on the central board of SANA. This was seen as a classic example of how nurses allowed the political agenda to entrench government policies in their profession.

The broader apartheid legislation of the country impacted in unison with the Nursing Act on the psyche of nurses. There were oppressive laws such as Pass laws, Influx Control, and the Group Areas Act. Nurse's lives at the micro-social level were hugely affected by legislation.

It should be underscored that the Nursing Act with all its amendments, further served to ensure the survival of whites as the masters.

Curriculum

The curriculum is geared to theoretical bulk and cannot develop critical thinking. Besides the formal aspect there is a hidden curriculum. This means that what you learn in the classroom is linked to what you talk about in the Nurses Home. That is all part of the socialisation process.

Oppression is perpetuated daily in the curriculum. A graphic example of the use of undemocratic methods is not having students determine their learning objectives. Another example is not allowing for group work.

Furthermore nursing education and nursing practice is based on Christian Philosophy, as though it was preordained for nurses to be *humble in spirit*, and not to question things. In the Eurocentric context, their options for participation, for practice is cut down.
The most familiar dictum is: "Ours is not to reason why, ours is but to do or die".

Classism

The wearing of epaulettes is seen as a divisive factor. It carries oppression within the ranks and affects the relationship of nurses to other professions by creating a special "nurse" consciousness.

Unequal Power Relations

Politics was brought into nursing by the state. While the state was able to use force in the social arena to implement its policies, in nursing it was through SANC that mental suppression of nurses was ensured. Therefore the ultimate culprit was the state, using the SANC to control nurses through nursing education.

Unequal power relations were further entrenched by means of a vertical line in the hierarchy. The nurse at the bottom is powerless to make changes, similarly the one at the middle management level and ironically the one at the very top has to go to a medical superintendent or medical director.

Mechanisms Used to Oppress

Apart from the curriculum the following mechanisms were incorporated into daily routines:

Language:
Wherever Afrikaans prevailed as a regional language, orders were given in Afrikaans, whether understood or not.

Nepotism:
This was used to entrench white superiority. White nurses had upward mobility, not granted to Black nurses, and higher salaries that did not relate directly to their qualifications, or workload, when compared to those of the Black nurses.

Doctor-domination:
The handmaiden role expected by doctors and the gender oppression emanating from them deprived nurses of freedom and participation. Under the medical model the nursing profession is unable to stand for *independent functions.*

Routine:
Nurses often encounter medical malpractice during routine work such as the giving out of medicines. Over-prescription is a medical mistake that nurses often need to correct.

Para-professionals such as physiotherapists, radiographers, etc have an unfavourable perception of nurses. For example, they would expect the nurse to lift a patient whereas, once the patient is handed over, it becomes their responsibility to lift and turn.

Professor Eric Mafune, at the time was in the Human Resource division at Wits University emphasised, in a workshop, that mental liberation entails change of attitude within the individual.

"If you don't challenge routine, you have never been proactive, you never asked, "How can I make a difference?" He admonished nurses not to stereotype them selves, never to settle for a comfortable routine.

LAHLEKILE

CONCLUSION

The Cutting Edge.

Much has changed since we entered the new millennium. An explosion of motivational material indicates that society is moving away from materialism and the domination of science, in the direction of spiritual evolution. That is the good news.

However, the environment is changing too, and humankind finds itself on the cusp of survival. The obstacles to survival are monumental. Poverty is here to stay. Even though efforts are being made to overcome the disparity between rich and poor, human greed and globalisation are making an impact. Other threats include genetically engineered foods, the increasing threat of a Third World War, increased violence against women and girls in times of peace, and the rise of fundamentalism. The latter is perceived by the world's feminist movement as 'the greatest threat to women in the modern world.'

In relation to these dangers we cannot avoid the question – what is happening in the nursing profession now that we are at the cutting edge of the new millennium?

A positive political atmosphere has been achieved in South Africa owing to the marvellous constitution, and it is reasonable to expect that similarly, a positive milieu exists for nurses with the demise of the former nursing associations. So let us ask introspectively, 'What has changed?'

It would seem that on the individual front, South African nurses have discovered the pot-of-gold their older counterparts have been hankering after. Only, it is not at the end of a rainbow. Currently, countries such as Britain and Saudi Arabia are vigorously recruiting our nurses.

This is not the first exodus of nurses. In the 1970s large numbers flocked to northern countries and to Australia. What is different now is that the pendulum has swung and democracy is no longer a pipe dream.

The current brain drain of nurses needs to be looked at closely, to the point of public dialogue. Issues raised here are of crucial importance. It should be of concern to DENOSA to research the current exodus of nurses to foreign soil. At the same time it offers a rich field for academics to explore.

What has the Government done to hold on to its nursing personnel? Is remuneration the only reason why nurses are departing from our shores? After all, salaries have been democratised as long as twelve to fourteen years ago. Furthermore, in democratic times, there have been 'adjustments' under fierce union pressure. Sadly for nurses, these adjustments are not market-related.

This is precisely why the private sector is able to siphon off trained nurses. They are able to pay better salaries and why is this? It is simply because they do not have the burden of having to provide nursing education. Government spends approximately R400, 000 to educate one nurse across four years, owing to the nursing student being an employee and at the same time having access to other benefits, such as medical aid or even a housing subsidy in some cases.

However, once training is over, nurses are floated free to join the ranks of the unemployed until they secure posts for themselves. There is despondency in the nursing world owing to the lack of posts or existing posts being 'frozen'. Nor are there any career prospects for nurses. As a consequence, nursing agencies are able to exploit this gap even though nursing education is not energised by the private sector.

Another factor is that nurses do not enjoy equity along with doctors and pharmacists. The Department of Health has opened up one year for doctors and pharmacists to gain experience in practice. A professional Health Council was envisaged for three categories of health care providers: doctors, nurses and pharmacists, but this has not yet materialised. It ought to be challenged by the nursing authorities. Failure to succeed in establishing a council is an indication that nursing does not have equity.

In the Eastern Cape, there are scores of unskilled people employed within the provincial Department of Health. This stems from the "inheritance" of two homelands, Ciskei and Transkei. They comprise laundry workers, labourers, and gardeners. Labour Relations apathy further compounds the problem of a bloated civil service.

Attempts were made to cut down drastically the numbers of support staff. When severance packages became available however, it was not this segment that snatched at the packages, but rather many of the civil servants, moreover those in decision-making positions.

People on the ground found it extremely difficult to understand why posts were frozen and why the persistent response of Government to salary demands was a 'lack of money'.

A further deflection of Government finance in 'the poorest province' occurred when the 'consultants' entered the equation. Not only did they join the civil servants at the financial trough, they actually siphoned off millions of the fiscal budget and were able to enrich themselves in this way. Some of these consultants were nurses. One or two seemed to be in permanent employment.

The nursing profession contains the skills base for health care delivery. Yet at the start of the new millennium, nothing moves. There are no promotions, no nursing leadership in sight, and no career prospects. What lies over the profession, like impenetrable fog, is a general feeling of despondency. Even should the management staff-load be increased for nurses, this does not increase the human resource element on the ground. Equipment is not being purchased, hospitals are not being maintained.

Nurses desire to work in an environment conducive to health, and they are able to experience this in the private sector or by working in other countries. In the public sector of their own land, nothing has happened for them. Wide-scale corruption within departments and rising state bankruptcy has impacted negatively on nursing. And it is not only nurses who are leaving, but also pharmacists, doctors and teachers.

LAHLEKILE

I believe that the situation is graver than is presently realized. If this chronicle would end on an honest note, then Lahlekile has to conclude with these words:

The political struggle of nursing is not over. Who will write Patekile and when?

REFERENCES

1. Women and Health in Africa, edited by Meredith Turshen, Africa World Press Inc. New Jersey, 1991. NURSING IN SOUTH AFRICA: BLACK WOMEN ORGANISE: NONCEBA LUBANGA

2. The Mind of South Africa 1990, Allistair Sparks, William Heineman Ltd.

3. The History of Medical Missions in South Africa, Christian Doctor and Nurse 1984, M. Gelfund. Publishied by the Aitken family and friends 93 East Avenue, Atholl-Sandton 2169, R.S.A.

4. Three Addresses to the Ciskei Mission Council [reprinted from the South African Outlook] 1940 NATIVE HEALTH Neil Mac vicar MD, DPH, Rev. H.M. Bennet MB, CLB., Dr. Dorothy Ryan. The Lovedale press.

5. Die Ou Man in Kettings 1988, Vier Swart Verhale: GELIFDE MOEDER. At Van Wyk, Uitgegee deur Saayman en Weber [ED ms] Bpk.

6. Standard Encyclopedic Dictionary: Funk and Wagnalls.

7. Tribute to Sister Dora, 1991 for Weekend Post by Jenny Cullum

8. Nursing in Society, 1978, Dolan, Josephine. W.B. Saunders Company

9. Lovedale Press Collection, Register of Documents No.28 1994. Cory Library for Historical Research. Rhodes University Grahamstown. Register edited by S.C.T. Fold

10. The History of the Development of Nursing in South Africa 1652-1960 by Charlotte Searle, 1965. The South African Nursing Association, Pretoria.

11. The Weekly Mail and Guardian: June 10-16 1994, pg 6-7.

12. Living Magazine, January 1994. Article on Witchcraft by Guy Hobbs.

13. An Historical Overview of Nursing Struggles in South Africa: CRITICAL HEALTH No.24, November 1998

14. CECELIA MAKIWANE: The Last Year, SANA Journal, June, 1977.

15. Register for Nurses and Midwives: 1st January 1949. Published by the SANC [Nursing Council] in terms of The Nursing Act No.45 of 1944

16. Marionhill: A Study of Bantu Life and Missionary Effort. Published by Marionhill Mission Press.

17. The Study of District Six Past and Present. Edited by Shamil Jeppe and Crain Soudien for

the "Hands off District Six" Committee 1990, published by Buchu Books.

REFERENCE PICTURES

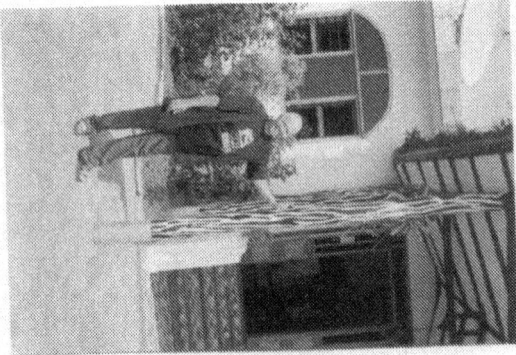

Gender activism in Uganda 2001

J0001

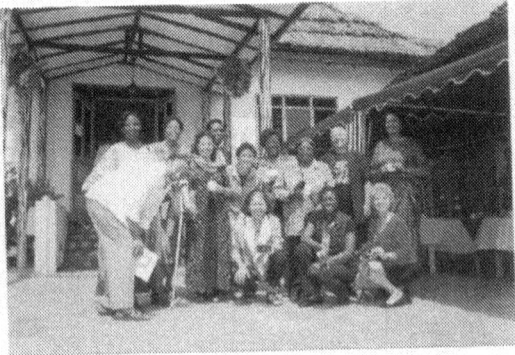

J0002

Front left : Dr Nadia Tubcaz, founder of Amanitare
Back : 2nd from right, Doreen, with the pioneers
of Amanitare.

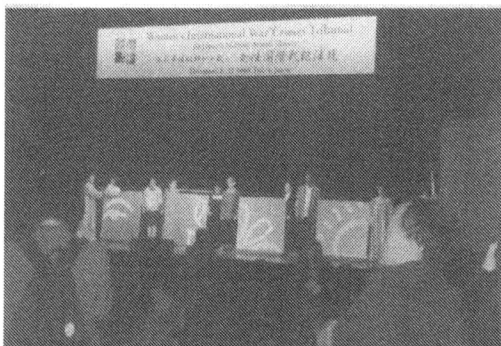

10005

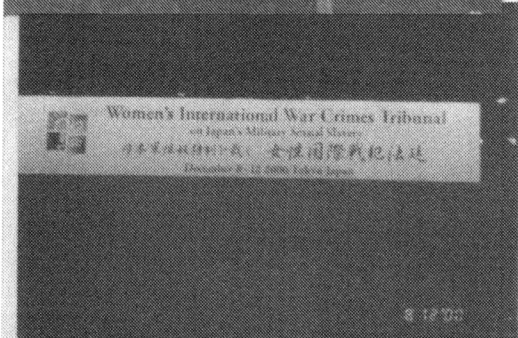

10006

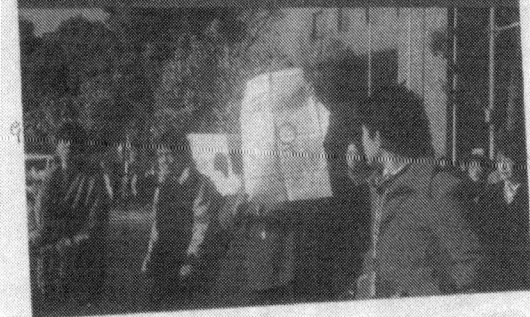

10007

LAHLEKILE

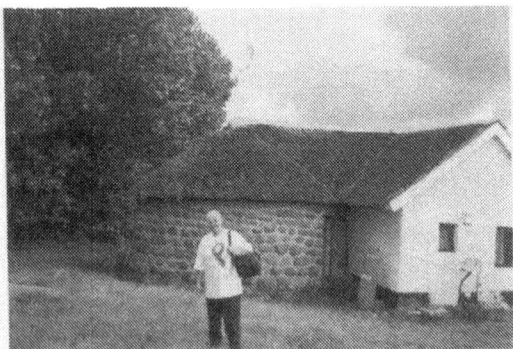

10004

Lesotho court
Residence in the Lesotho court, high up on the mountainside
on the property of a mission hospital

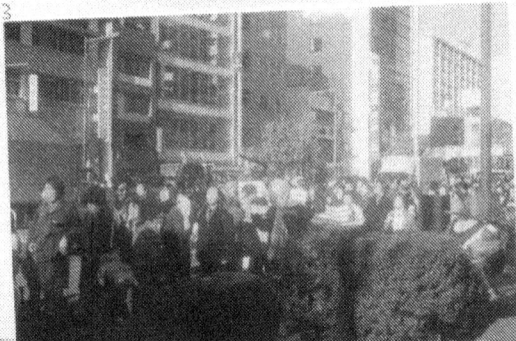

10003

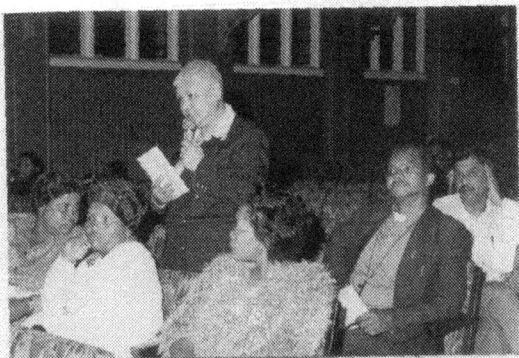

10010: An activist in Action, Doreen with Mike

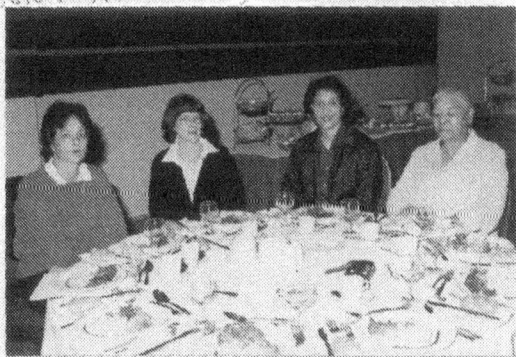

10011: Women's day Dinner. Doreen right.

LAHLEKILE

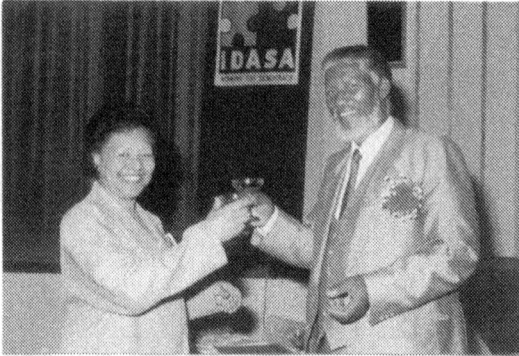

Prior to the first historical Nurses' Conference:
Mr Tyatywa ... [then] chairman of DASAN — is the
Democratic Association of SA Nurses ... and
Doreen ..... [then] Secretary of DASAN.

* DASAN and CONSA [Congress of Nurses of SA]
pioneered the running of the first of three
national nursing conferences.

10008

10012- Local Launch or Lanbekile

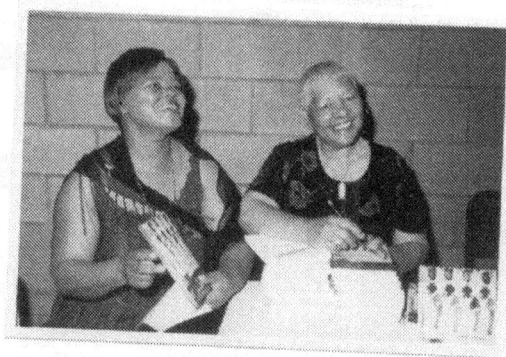

LAHLEKILE

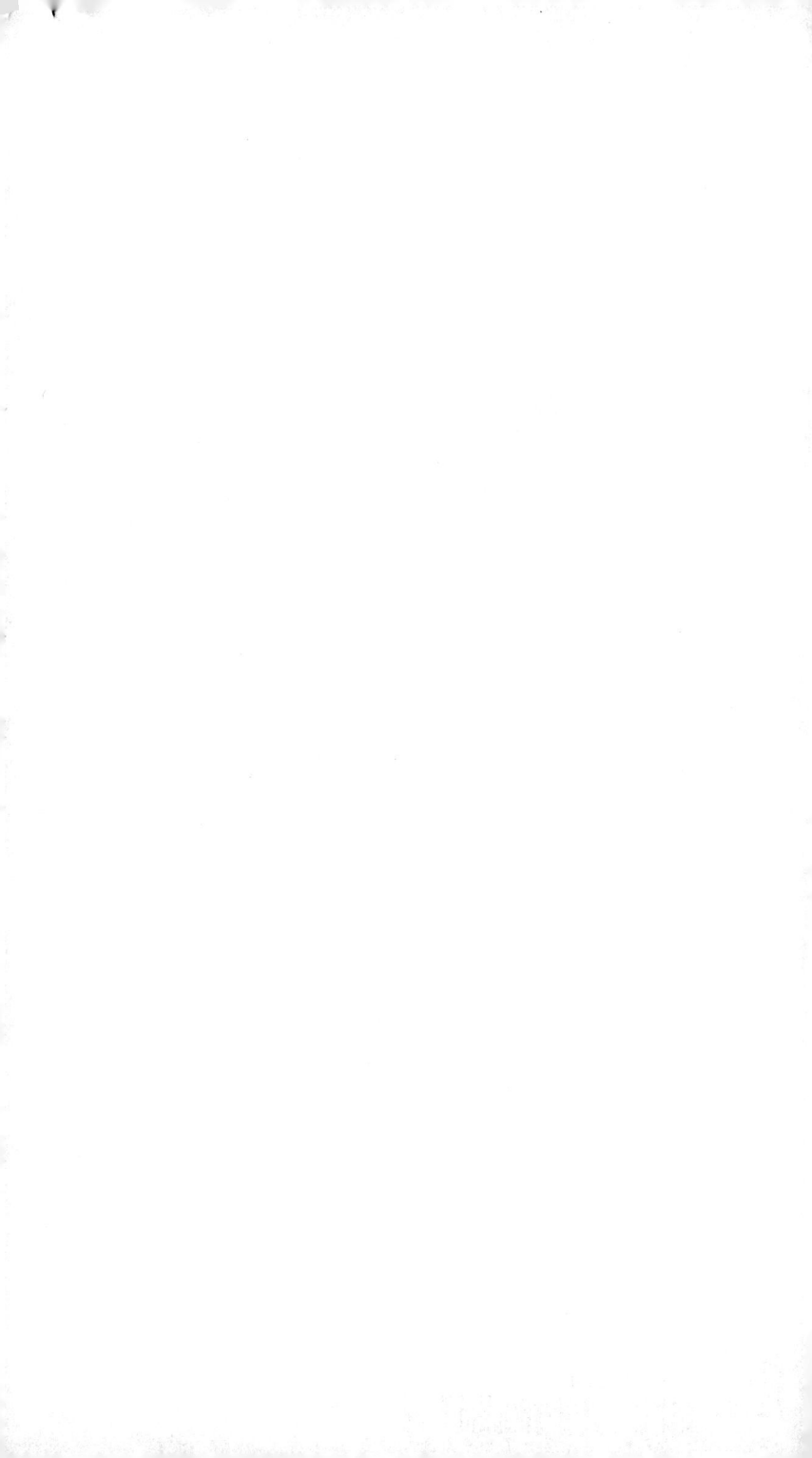

www.ingramcontent.com/pod-product-compliance
Lightning Source LLC
Chambersburg PA
CBHW020603270326
41927CB00005B/150